Outdoorsman's Fitness and Medical Guide

Outdoorsman's

Fitness
and Medical
Guide

By Lawrence Galton

Drawings by Tom Beecham

OUTDOOR LIFE · HARPER & ROW · NEW YORK

Contents

Outdoorsman's Fitness and Medical Guide

Part I

PREPARING FOR OUTDOOR TRIPS

1 Physical Fitness and the Outdoorsman

Whatever your favorite outdoor activity, you can multiply your enjoyment of it by getting into top physical shape. Let's face it: Hunting, fishing, virtually every enjoyable outdoor sport calls for physical exertion—sometimes, vigorous exertion. Nobody would want it any other way.

But no man, however good his general health and his experience and skill as an outdoorsman, can lead a more or less sedentary existence during most of the year and then take off, without penalty, chasing game through muskeg or heavy foliage, scrambling through broken, mountainous country, crawling on his belly, or riding a horse from dawn to dusk on a pack trip. Every year, some hunters die of heart attacks because they aren't in condition for a vigorous hunt. For millions of others, the excitement of the sport is dulled by exhaustion.

Despite the best equipment and the most careful plans, there can be misery for the physically unprepared in backpacking, snow camping, paddling and portaging a canoe, and other activities that call for strength in muscles rarely put to rough test at other times.

The fact is that most of us today, on the job and off,

lead soft lives. Progress—represented by power tools and automation, elevators and cars, TV sets and electric toothbrushes—contributes to an ever-growing reduction of physical expenditures.

Even the man whose job calls for a moderate amount of physical activity and who, in addition, is active on weekend fishing, hunting or camping trips, is far from being in peak shape.

You can't get into top condition overnight. But if you have no serious physical defects, you can, within a reasonable time, develop the strength and stamina to enjoy every outdoor trip, get more out of it than possibly you have ever gotten before.

In at least one sense, the human body is like a car. Drive a car at its top speed—say 120 miles an hour—and you expect it to burn more gas per mile than at 60, well below its peak capacity. So with the body. Push up its capacity and thereafter, working well below the peak, you get high efficiency—more work done with relatively less energy expenditure.

By increasing capacity, you develop reserves for the toughest stresses—for the sudden and unexpected, for feats of strength you otherwise couldn't achieve. And, more than that, you greatly increase your efficiency for the routine.

Many scientific studies have been showing recently that it is never too late to improve on physical condition. In some particularly notable research carried out at the Civil Aeromedical Research Institute of the Federal Aviation Agency in Norman, Oklahoma, Dr. Bruno Balke checked hundreds of men in the age range from 17 to 65 years. He found that physical working capacity was "by no means related to the process of growing older in years; professors surpassed young students, staff officers outperformed basic trainees. It all seemed to depend upon the regular activity level people usually are engaged in."

His investigations showed that even with thirty to forty minutes a day of the simplest kind of exercise—alternate trotting and walking—middle-aged men with sedentary living habits could improve their capacities by 25 percent in ten weeks.

Balke's studies even covered a group of patients hospitalized with chronic lung disease. It takes some energy expenditure just to maintain breathing, circulation and body temperature in the resting state in bed. This is called basal metabolic rate. With a simple fitness program, the patients in a short time were able to increase their energy expenditure capacity to six times the basal metabolic rate.

Another interesting finding coming out of the studies has to do with what fraction of the body's physical capacity can be used without undue stress in daily work. Experiments showed that well-trained people could tolerate a 50 percent load occasionally for ten to twelve hours; they could work at half their "rated peak capacity" for that long. And, without undue strain, they could take a 33 percent load for eight to ten hours a day for several consecutive days. On the other hand, untrained people had to quit under a 33 percent load after just three to four hours because of exhaustion.

With an intelligently executed program to improve physical fitness, you can expect many dividends in everyday life as well as when you're in the field. Beyond firming flabby muscles, research has been showing, a fitness program can improve efficiency of heart, lungs and circulation. Overall body, not just individual muscle, strength increases; endurance goes up; flexibility and coordination increase. End results include general improvement in health and increased ability to carry on sustained effort and resist fatigue—and tension.

Fitness, Fatigue and Tension

Emotional tension and chronic fatigue are among the most common complaints today. Even some years ago, a distinguished researcher, Dr. Peter Karpovich, Professor of Physiology at Springfield College, was reporting that the human body has a capacity for generating 14 horsepower with maximum exertion while it generates only 0.1 horsepower at rest.

In many who lead sedentary lives the unused horsepower may well go into building up tension—with the tension then becoming involved in producing fatigue and sometimes other complaints as well.

Typical of many cases to be found in recent medical reports is that of a man in his late thirties who, after having moved up far in his career, should have been at the height of his powers. Instead, he complained of sleeping problems, chronic fatigue, increasing difficulty in concentrating effectively on his work and in handling matters he once could take care of with little effort. He suffered from frequent headaches and a variety of vague complaints that made him feel always under par. Although his blood pressure was up a little, tests disclosed no disease. The prescription: a progressive program of activity to build up his physical fitness. No medicine.

Within a few months, he was sleeping well, felt relaxed and vigorous. His blood pressure was down. He was turning out better work in less time, finding time to get outdoors, and having more fun than he'd had since college days.

Fitness and the Heart

It used to be thought that exercise was bad for the heart. One research project after another has been showing that this is not necessarily so.

In the summer of 1965, a team of American scientists made a special trip to study Masai tribesmen in Africa, trying to discover why these herdsmen and warriors never seem to get heart trouble despite a diet containing enough cholesterol to send the ordinary worried American fleeing in panic from the dinner table.

The Masai live almost exclusively on meat and on milk with a butterfat content that soars to about 6.5 percent. Yet they have far lower blood cholesterol levels on the average than do Americans.

Evidently, it's exercise that protects Masai hearts, keeps cholesterol levels in their blood low despite the high dietary intake. The Masai are known to walk as much as fifty to sixty miles a day—and to do it without strain.

The scientists brought along a treadmill designed to move at a speed of 1½ miles per hour and to tilt progressively upward at the front end one degree every minute so that it becomes increasingly difficult to keep walking and even stay on the mill.

An average healthy American college boy lasts fourteen minutes before being spilled off the back end, exhausted and gasping for breath. The average Masai—and the group of thirty-nine taking the test included a number of old men—lasted twenty-three minutes and not one sat down after his performance. Two of the men walked the treadmill right off its maximum scale of thirty minutes and 30-degree elevation.

The Boston Irishmen and the Irish Irishmen

Recently Harvard scientists compared 700 Boston Irishmen with their brothers who stayed in Ireland. Coronary heart disease deaths in the Boston group (ages 30 to 60) were two times those in the Ireland group. The men in Ireland ate more eggs, more butter and more other saturated fats—yet had lower serum cholesterol levels. They consumed 400 calories more per day than their Boston counterparts but weighed 10 percent less.

Says Dr. Frederick J. State of Harvard: "The men in Ireland were getting more exercise and their lower cholesterol levels show that physical activity is more than just burning off calories."

At a special Conference on Preventive Cardiology at the University of Vermont not long ago, physician investigators stressed that the prophylactic value of regular physical activity has received too little attention. They pointed out that the trained heart beats slowly, functions more economically, requires less oxygen for a given amount of work. In addition, the well-exercised body requires a smaller amount of heart muscle activity for a given physical performance than the untrained body.

As they put it in somewhat technical language: "These combined effects of training reduce the demands on coronary blood supply and, together with an improved development of collaterals (extra branch blood vessels to feed the heart muscle), protect the heart against myocardial ischemia (blood starvation) even in the presence of some degree of coronary stenosis (artery narrowing)."

Revitalizing the Heart

Says Dr. Harry Johnson of the Life Extension Foundation in New York: "In the thirty years between 1930 and 1960, deaths from coronary heart disease increased 2000 percent. It was during this same thirty years that we started to drive rather than walk—that suburban communities were laid out without sidewalks—that a man walking down the street became a subject of investigation by the police—that the only exercise in golf was extracted by the invention of the electric golf cart."

Adds Johnson: "We forget the heart thrives on work. It pumps to circulate blood. If the blood has difficulty in getting through, as in coronary heart disease, new blood vessels will push through to keep the muscle supplied with blood. Regular exercise, by keeping the circulatory system in shape, can help prevent blockage of the arteries."

Dr. Johnson tells of a laborer who died of an accident in his sixties. "An autopsy revealed that earlier in his life the main coronary artery of his heart was blocked. But because he was always a vigorous man, collateral circulation (extra blood vessels) was developed to supply the heart muscle with blood. Without exercise, he would probably have been dead before fifty."

Bringing Down the Pressure

The value of exercise in combating not only high blood cholesterol but also high blood pressure and over-weight, two other factors believed to be involved in setting the stage for heart attacks, has been shown in a recent study at Vanderbilt University.

Vanderbilt investigators worked with a group of men, 21 to 40 years of age, all with at least one of the heart attack factors present, some with two and even three. For six weeks, the men were put through a physical conditioning program that began with mild exercises and built up to mile runs and fast sprints. By the end of the six-week program, they had lost an average of 6 pounds each and both serum cholesterol and blood pressure levels were significantly lower.

Some physicians now believe that high cholesterol level in the blood usually is not associated with coronary artery disease unless another blood fat, triglyceride, also is elevated. And exercise can reduce the triglyceride level, a University of Illinois study has shown.

Fifteen professional men, ranging in age from 35 to 55, were put through a course of physical conditioning. One already had had a heart attack nine months before. In the beginning, the mean triglyceride level in the fifteen men was almost 50 percent above the upper limit of normal. As the result of exercise it fell to 10 percent below upper normal.

Recently, the American Medical Association took a hard, long look at physical fitness and concluded:

"Belief in the healthfulness of regular, suitable exercise, previously based on tradition and logic, is constantly being bolstered by evidence from research . . .

"Studies of the life histories of those who maintain a relatively higher degree of fitness through the nature of their work or through other activities seem to indicate that they suffer less degenerative disease and probably live longer than those who follow a sedentary life."

They are also likely to lead more rewarding lives. And there is certainly that promise for the man who loves his outdoor jaunts and can expect, when he is in top shape for them, to get far more unadulterated pleasure out of them.

2 Understanding Your Body

Getting into top form isn't a matter of working out to increase the size and power of a few obvious muscles. It's a help in understanding what you need to do for sound fitness if you have a clear picture of certain basic aspects of body physiology.

Muscles

Better than half the human body is made up of muscles. There are more than 600, which play a role in everything we do. They suck air into the lungs, push food through the digestive tract, as well as account for every motion.

Each muscle is composed of a bundle of fibers. Each fiber is roughly about the size of a human hair yet can support 1,000 times its own weight. All told, there are some 6 trillion muscle fibers in the body.

Each muscle works by contraction, shortening by as much as one-third to one-half. And the contraction—which can take place in a few thousandths of a second as, for example, with the twitch of an eyelid—is the result of a complex series of chemical events.

Muscles themselves are built up from amino acids, materials derived from protein foods. They are fueled by fats and a starch, glycogen, which the body derives from the diet.

During strenuous activity, not enough oxygen may be available for the complete combustion of the fats and glycogen. Lactic acid is formed, accumulates in the muscles and causes fatigue.

During a sprint, for example, a runner may actually need several times as much oxygen as his body can provide immediately. Muscles can adapt to continuing their work without the full quota of oxygen—for a limited period. An "oxygen debt" is built up, and after the race the runner breathes hard for a time until the debt is paid off.

The better trained the body is, the longer before the debt begins to build up—and the quicker the recovery, too. The reason lies in circulatory efficiency.

The Circulation

Muscles are provisioned with food and oxygen, and their wastes are carried off, through thousands of miles of hairlike capillaries.

Fresh blood moves out from the heart through the body's major trunkline, the aorta, which splits into branches that run to various areas. In turn, the branches split into lesser branches which split still more, finally forming capillaries. Of the total 70,000 miles of blood vessels in the body, the capillaries make up the largest proportion. Their volume is great enough to hold the body's entire blood supply of about 5 quarts.

But only part of the capillary system has blood flowing through it at any moment. The capillaries are designed to open and close under the direction of nerves which exert their control in response to demand. When muscles are not used, they have relatively little need for blood and nourishment and most of the capillaries supplying them remain collapsed, out of business most of the time. The greater the activity of muscles—and need for blood—the more the capillaries open up and, in fact, the more capillaries may be developed to supply the need. With sedentary living, there is little demand.

One famed experiment by Dr. Hardin Jones of the University of California has shown that the average sedentary American man is, in terms of muscle circulation, middle-aged by the time he is 26. Using Geiger counter tests to follow blood flow through muscles in teen-agers and in 500 industrial workers, Dr. Jones established that between the age of 18 and the age of 25, the flow drops 40 percent; by the age of 35, it's down 60 percent, at which point, in the sense of physical vigor, the average sedentary man is less than half the man he used to be.

The Goals for Fitness

Pure muscle size isn't a true measure of fitness for anybody—and it's least of all what the outdoorsman wants. The objectives of a well-founded training program should be to strengthen muscles and also the circulatory system which provides for endurance—the ability to sustain activity and keep going without quick fatigue when you're in the field and the ability, too, every day, to get your work done and have energy left over.

When you're at rest all the muscles in the body use only about 1/30 of the oxygen they can use during maximum effort. With a well-rounded, progressive program of exercise, they can be made to use still more. When they do, the heart will respond, pumping harder to get more oxygen-carrying blood into circulation, and, over a period of time, heart pumping efficiency will increase; the heart will pump more blood with each stroke.

At the same time, lung capacity—much of it never used in sedentary living—will enlarge to absorb and feed more oxygen into the blood stream. The higher oxygen content will aid muscle nutrition.

As circulation improves both in quality and quantity throughout the body, the capillaries penetrating into muscles will open wider and become more effective.

The total effect is admirable: Muscles are strengthened; so is the whole supporting system. You build endurance along with power. Muscles can do more work and more powerful work—and can do it longer without fatigue. If you build up an oxygen debt after a particularly strenuous bit of work in the field or anywhere else, it's paid off more quickly. If you tire, you recover more quickly.

Basic Principles

Achieving these objectives isn't a matter of rushing off to a gym and knocking yourself out lifting weights, or going all-out for handball or basketball, or indiscriminately undertaking some variety of calisthenics.

Go and lift 200 pounds over your head and if you haven't done it before it may be your last act on earth. Take on a daily routine of some mild setting up exercises and you'll undoubtedly feel a bit better—but hardly toughened up for a vigorous outdoor life.

What's needed is a program that follows certain key principles.

First is "tolerance." There should be no sudden call on your body for a burst of tremendous effort. Excessive straining beyond the level your bodily functions are ready to handle isn't necessary at the beginning or at any time. It can produce injuries.

Second is "overload." An easy workout will not improve you very much. You have to push yourself a bit, work harder than you usually do in the normal day's activities, and work beyond the first feeling of tiredness. But all this still within your tolerance limits. In effect, you are not overloading your body. It has more capacity than it is ordinarily called upon to use. You give it a bit more load than usual—and it can handle it. Progressively, it will be able to handle more.

"Progression" is the third cardinal principle. As you maintain a regular schedule of exercise and your strength and endurance grow, your workouts, if unmodified, will become easier and easier for you and you will reach a plateau. You will have improved. With the same workouts, you will maintain the improvement. To go beyond, you must make the workouts progressively more strenuous until you arrive at the level of fitness you want to achieve.

All of these principles are incorporated in the workouts in the following pages. The chapters that follow in this section on fitness provide a basic progressive training program and additional suggestions for the outdoorsman.

The basic program. It's designed to allow you to start at your present level of fitness and progressively work up to higher and higher levels—as high as you want to go. All of the exercises can be done in and around the home. They require time—but little equipment. They are well-rounded, designed for building both strength and endurance.

Jogging. Jogging today is becoming increasingly popular—deservedly. While it is not an essential part of the basic program, many outdoorsmen may be interested in it because of its endurance-increasing and other values. A chapter on jogging outlines these values and how, if you wish, you can use jogging in conjunction with the basic program.

Isometrics. Although isometric exercises have been overly touted as a means of building fitness in a few minutes a day, they cannot do that; but they do have values. A chapter showing how isometrics can be put to use is included.

You will also find in Chapter 6 some suggestions for further toughening up certain muscles you may be putting to strenuous use on particularly rugged trips.

Included, too, is a special chapter, "If Time is Short." The ideal fitness program is progressive, extended. But if, right now, you have a hunting, fishing or other trip all planned for a month from now, you will find a program in this chapter to help you get ready for the trip, to put you into as good shape as possible in a short time and to do it safely. When you return, you can pick up the basic program and, because of the special workouts and your activities on the trip, progress rapidly.

Wise First Step: A Medical Check

A physical examination at least once a year is advisable for everybody. If you haven't had one recently, it's a good idea to have your doctor check you over before you start training.

None of us ever can know precisely what's going on inside—state of the heart and of other organs and functions. To be free of symptoms doesn't necessarily mean to be in perfect health. Careful check-ups of men, both young and old, frequently turn up unsuspected problems—and very often they are still minor, readily remedied.

With an examination under your belt, you can confidently begin to get into top shape. Chances are your doctor will give you a hearty O.K. If you should have some problem, he may well have suggestions for modifying your program to make it more beneficial for you.

3 The Progressive Fitness Program

The program in this chapter provides a series of exercises that will take you progressively from your present level of fitness to as high a level as you wish to go.

Each workout is divided into three phases:

1. Warm-up
2. Strengthening and endurance-building calisthenics
3. A single continuous activity—one of a number from which you can choose—to further stimulate and strengthen circulatory and respiratory systems and add vigor.

Regularity is important. Work out as often as you can—five or six times a week if at all possible; if not, at least three. A once-a-week workout, however prolonged, is of little value.

There is no one "best" time of day for training. Just after meals isn't to be recommended but virtually any other time that is convenient is good. It could be early in the morning or the last thing before going to bed at night, not bad preparation for a good night's sleep. Also to be considered: after you get home from work, before dinner. You may well find that, far from leaving you tired, a workout at this time may refresh you.

FIRST MONTH

PHASE ONE—*The Warm-Up*

It's important to warm up gradually before working out hard. Light warm-up exercises not only limber up muscles; they also prepare the heart and lungs for exertion, give them a chance to get ready to function more effectively. At the same time, they serve to tune up the central nervous system. The fact is that when you move one muscle, another muscle, the antagonist of the first, should relax its tension properly. The nervous system controls this.

Warming up also is a safety measure. As one physician puts it: "After taxiing his plane out to the runway, a pilot stops, guns up each motor in turn, checks response to controls. By simulated load conditions, he is bringing components up to optimum temperature and pressure ranges. Such a routine seems to be an obvious safety measure. The warm-up in similar fashion is concerned with safety features."

While there continues to be some controversy among coaches as to whether a warm-up ever actually improves athletic performance, there is evidence it helps reduce risk of injury—in a race, a ballgame and during exercise.

You'll be using the following set of five warm-up exercises throughout—at the beginning of each workout.

They're not strenuous. And they don't take long. As you get into better and better shape, you can cut down a bit on them—but it's advisable not to stop entirely.

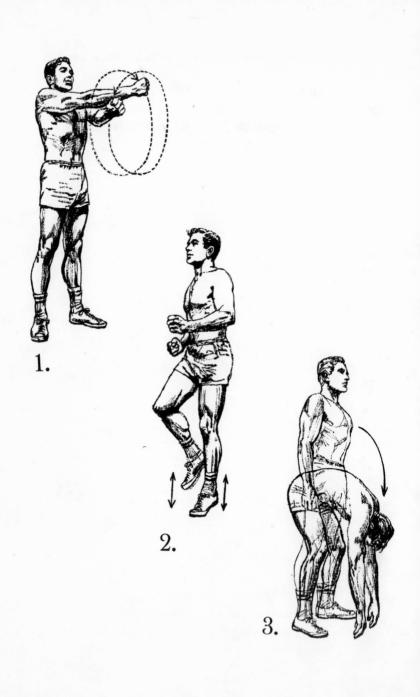

1.

2.

3.

1. Standing erect, swing your arms in circles, crisscrossing them in front of the body. About 30 seconds of this.

2. Run in place and breathe deeply. Raise each foot 4 or 5 inches off the floor. Count each time your right foot touches the floor. Run for a count of 100.

3. From erect position, feet 18 to 24 inches apart, hands at sides, stretch forward and down. Letting knees bend a little, slowly touch fingers to floor, and return to starting position. Repeat 10 times.

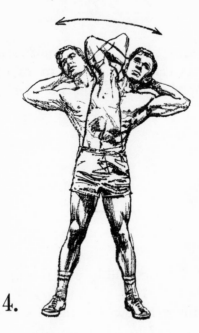

4.

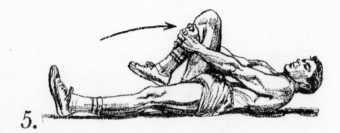

5.

4. Stand erect, feet 18 to 24 inches apart, hands behind the head, and gently bend upper part of body first to left, then to right. Repeat 10 times.

5. Lie flat on your back. Bend one leg, bring it up until you can reach it with both hands and grasp it below the knee, then gently bring it back some more, stretching both the leg and your arms. Do the same with the other leg. Repeat 6 times with each leg.

PHASE TWO

After starting each workout with the warm-up series, continue on to the eight exercises for Phase Two. They bring into play important muscle groups all over the body, some of which you use to some extent in daily activities, all of which you may call upon when you go off on an outdoor expedition.

If, at the beginning, you can't keep up an exercise for the time period shown, don't overstrain. Continue it as long as you can, take a few deep breaths, and go on to the next exercise.

You'll progress from workout to workout as you become able to:

(1) do all the exercises more easily, including any that may have been particularly difficult to begin with;

(2) accomplish more repetitions of the individual exercises in the given time periods; and

(3) go from one exercise to the next with less and less pause between.

Comparisons

Fitness is an individual matter. The best evaluation of your progress will be not in terms of how you compare with anybody else in ability to do the exercises but in how you keep improving your own record, how much better you feel every day and how much more you can enjoy yourself when you get out into the field.

Still, if you're interested in making some comparisons, you can make use of standards employed by the Navy and Marine Corps. They take into account age.

Thus, for example, for a man under 40, 20 to 24 situps per minute constitute satisfactory performance by Navy-Marine standards; 25 to 29, good; 30–35, excellent; 36 and more, outstanding. For a man over 40, 16 to 20 per minute is satisfactory performance; 21–24, good: 25–29, excellent; 30 and more, outstanding.

For pushups, for ages under 40, 15 to 16 per minute make a satisfactory performance; 17–19, good; 20–24, excellent; 25 and more, outstanding. If you're over 40, you're doing satisfactorily, by Navy-Marine standards, with 13–14 a minute; good with 15–17; excellent with 18–20; outstanding with 21 or more.

Good Signs and Bad

It's important never to overdo a workout. Take it easy at the outset of this program and make your workouts just a little more strenuous each time. Gradual progression will actually be progression; overdoing may only interrupt the progression, require a layoff period, even make you lose some ground.

If you step up the pace a little in each successive workout—and each time recover quickly afterward—it's a good sign. On the other hand, if you still notice several minutes after finishing a workout that you're breathless and your heart is pounding, or if you feel unduly weak or tired after a two-hour period, or notice definite and undue fatigue next day, then it's very likely you're overdoing, going beyond what you're ready and able to do at this stage of your training and strength.

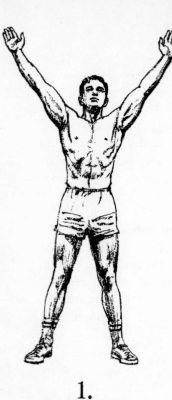

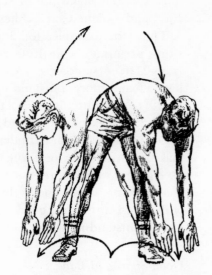

1.

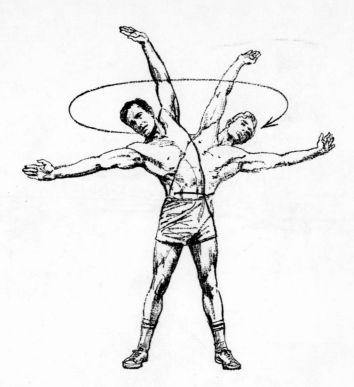

First Month—Phase Two

1. BENDS—2 minutes

Stand erect, feet 18 to 24 inches astride, hands overhead. Keeping knees straight, bend forward and down to touch the floor with fingers of both hands—first, outside the left foot, then between the feet, finally outside the right foot. Return to upright position. Then, with hands stretched overhead, bend the upper part of the body around in as big a circle as you can. Repeat for 2 minutes—as many times as you can.

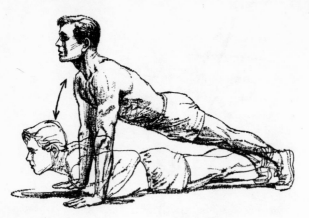

2.

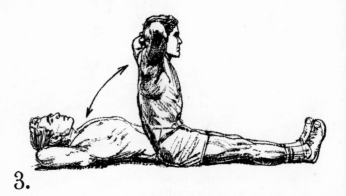

3.

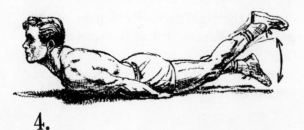

4.

2.   PUSHUPS—1 minute
Do full-length pushups as shown. Start
with chest on floor, hands directly under
shoulders, back and legs straight. Repeat
as many times as possible for one minute.
NOTE: If you're not able at first to perform pushups with legs straight, do them
from the knees until you can move onto
the full-length.

3.   SITUPS—1 minute
Lie on your back, arms clasped behind
head. Sit up, keeping feet on floor. Return
to original position. Repeat as often as possible in one minute. If necessary, to begin
with, you can hook feet under chair or sofa.

4.   FLUTTER KICK—1 minute
Lie on stomach, hands under thighs. Arch
back to bring chest and head up. Then
flutter kick. Keep legs 8 to 10 inches apart;
move them from the hip with slight bend
in knees. Count each kick as one.

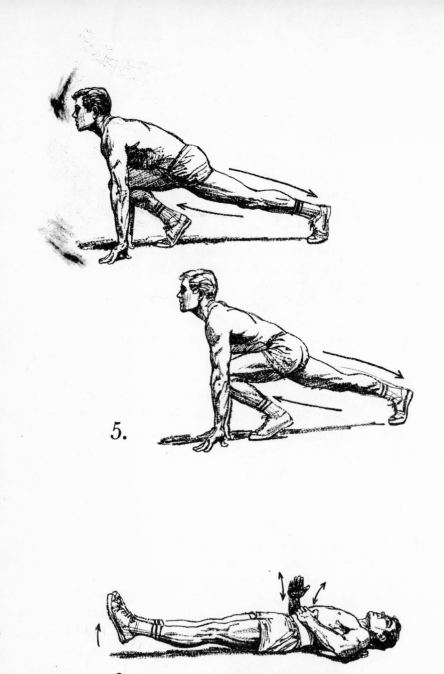

5.

6.

5. SPRINTING—1 minute
    Squat down, knees bent, hands on floor,
    fingers pointed ahead, with left leg ex-
    tended to rear. In one bouncing movement,
    reverse leg positions, bringing left foot up
    to hands, extending right leg to rear. Count
    one for each bounce. Repeat as often as
    you can for one minute.

6. SUSTAINED LEG RAISE—1 minute
    Lie on your back, raise both legs 4 to 5
    inches off the floor. Hold them there—up
    and steady—as long as you can, for the full
    minute if possible. At the same time, vigor-
    ously slap the abdomen, first with one
    hand, then with the other, continuing to
    breathe as deeply as you can.

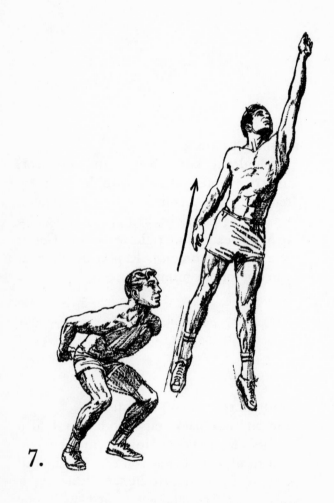

7.

7.   JUMP UP—1 minute
        Stand near a wall, bend knees, bring hands
        behind back, and position yourself for a
        leap upward. Then leap. Jump up as high
        as you can. Determine highest point you
        can reach, mark this lightly on the wall,
        then keep jumping, always trying to come
        within an inch of the high point. Repeat
        the jumps as often as possible in the one-
        minute period.

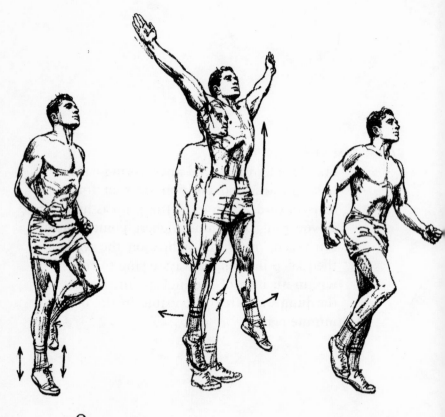

8.

8. STATIONARY RUN—6 minutes
Run in place, raising each foot at least 4 inches off floor. Each time right foot hits floor, count 1. After 100 counts, do 10 astride jumps as illustrated. Repeat running and jumping for 6 minutes.

PHASE THREE

By now you have spent several minutes warming up, another 14 minutes or so on Phase Two of your workout.

Take a few deep breaths and proceed to the third phase. This involves a single activity—one that calls for more energy expenditure and brings into play at once many different muscle groups and keeps them working longer than the individual exercises. The objective: to add still further to muscle strength, and also to endurance by stimulating and strengthening the circulatory and respiratory systems.

Walking

Walking is excellent. It's slow in terms of miles per hour; if you walk at the rate of 3 mph, you're moving. But it involves nearly all the muscles of the body, is universally available as an exercise nearly every day of the year. You can breathe deeply as you walk, exercising your lungs. The activity also promotes circulation. And you can readily regulate the strenuousness by pace and distance.

For the first month, an increasingly brisk mile walk will do well. If you can go beyond, achieve a very brisk mile and then add distance, fine.

Substitutes

Other activities can be substituted—provided they are continuous. Bicycling three to five miles, rowing a boat, swimming, playing handball or tennis—all are good.

Less to be preferred are such intermittent activities as bowling, golf. Increasingly popular and excellent as a phase three activity is jogging (See Chapter 4).

TAPERING OFF

No less important than warming up at the beginning of a workout is tapering off properly afterward. While you're actively exercising, the heart pumps out blood much faster than usual to keep the muscles supplied with oxygen and other nourishment. After carrying its supplies to the muscle tissues, the blood enters the vein system to return to the heart and lungs for fresh supplies. And, during exercise, the contracting muscles, by pressing on the veins, produce a kind of pumping action that helps get the blood back to heart and lungs.

If you stop exercising suddenly, the heart will continue for a while to pump extra blood but, with the muscles, especially those in the legs, no longer active, they no longer pump on the veins; and the extra supply, still being pumped by the heart, may pool in the muscles, causing a temporary shortage elsewhere in the body, making you feel faint, sometimes even making you pass out.

Also, it has been observed that cramps and stiffness are much more likely to develop when exercise is abruptly halted. A tapering off period can help prevent these discomforts.

To taper off, just keep moving about—in relaxed

fashion. Instead of plopping down in a chair, walk about, lazily bend and stretch as you walk, gently move your arms. A couple of minutes of this will do the job.

COOLING OFF

Don't rush into a hot tub or shower immediately after a workout—or even immediately after the tapering off period. Give yourself another two or three minutes to cool off. You need this period to radiate some of the heat you've worked up. If you jump right into or under hot water, your body temperature will still be above normal, the hot water will impede heat dissipation, and you'll come out of the bath still sweating.

Use these same rules for tapering and cooling off throughout this program.

PROGRESSION RECORD

If you'd like to keep a record of your progress as you work out during the first month, you can do so readily in the chart below.

Seven of the eight exercises in Phase Two call for as many repetitions as possible within given time periods. You can enter the repetitions you achieve. You can also note your time for the mile walk or make suitable entries for substitute activities.

You can make entries for each workout if you wish—although that is not essential. Recording your achievements for every third workout—or even for the final workout each week—will unmistakably show your progress.

PROGRESSION RECORD

EXERCISE	1st week	2nd week	3rd week	4th week
1				
2				
3				
4				
5				
6				
7				
8				
Mile Time				

SECOND MONTH

Now, after a month of working out, you undoubtedly can see and feel improvement. It takes time—there just are no shortcuts—to build up strength and endurance. And the amount of time required before the improvement becomes dramatic varies greatly from individual to individual, depending upon the level of fitness from which he started and the consistency of workouts.

If you're still not entirely comfortable with the exercises you've been using during the first month, stick with them until you are. In doing so, you will not be wasting time but will be making further progress.

If in your last few workouts, all has gone well and you got through them at a good pace, you're ready to move up to the next stage for progression.

PHASE ONE—*The Warm-Up*

The exercises here remain the same as for the first month (pages 22–24), since their purpose is strictly warm-up or get ready. You can continue them exactly as before, or it may be possible for you now to reduce the time or repetitions for each one by about one-third.

PHASE TWO

Five minutes longer are required for the Phase Two part of your workout now. There are nine exercises instead of eight. Some of the original eight remain as they were; for others, the time period is increased; and for still others, modifications are introduced.

Your workout now will be more demanding—but not too much so. The exercises are designed to keep up with your growing strength and endurance and to add to them in the only possible way—by calling for increasingly vigorous exertion.

Again the same rules apply. Don't go overboard. Take it easy at the outset. Try to step up the pace a little in each successive workout. If at any time you feel you've overdone—as indicated by failure to recover quickly after a workout, long continued breathlessness, fatigue next day—drop the pace well back for the next workout and thereafter increase it less rapidly.

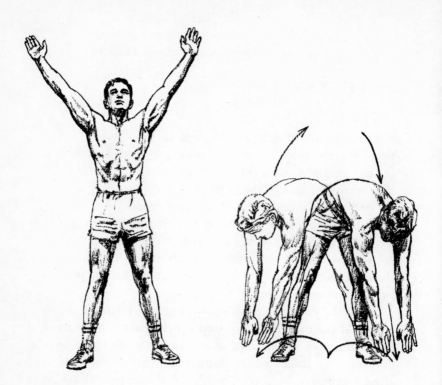

1.

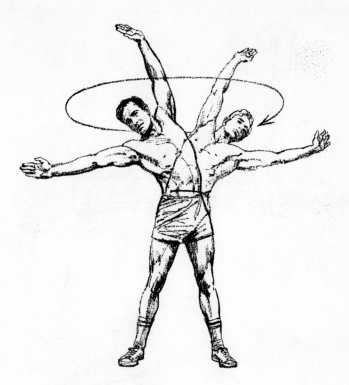

Second Month, Phase Two

1. BENDS—2 minutes

Stand erect, feet 18 to 24 inches apart, hands overhead. Keeping knees straight, bend forward and down to touch the floor with fingers of both hands—first, outside the left foot, then between the feet, finally outside the right foot. Return to upright position. Then, with hands stretched overhead, bend the upper part of the body around in as big a circle as you can. Repeat for 2 minutes, as often as you can.

2.

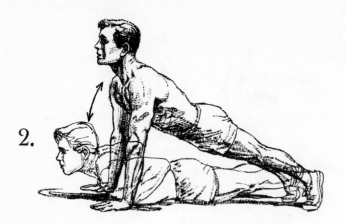

3.

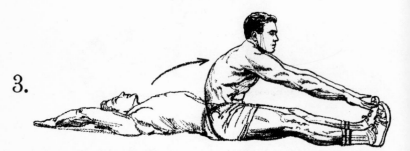

4.

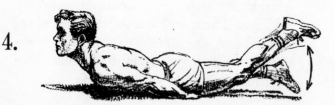

2. PUSHUPS—2 minutes

Do full-length pushups. Start with chest on floor, hands directly under shoulders, back and legs straight. Repeat as many times as possible in two minutes.

3. MODIFIED SITUPS—1 minute

Lie on your back, legs straight, feet together, arms straight out overhead. Sit up to touch the toes. Repeat as often as possible in one minute.

4. FLUTTER KICK—2 minutes

Lie on stomach, hands under thighs. Arch back to bring chest and head up. Then flutter kick. Keep legs 8 to 10 inches apart; move them from the hip with slight bend in knees. Count each kick as one.

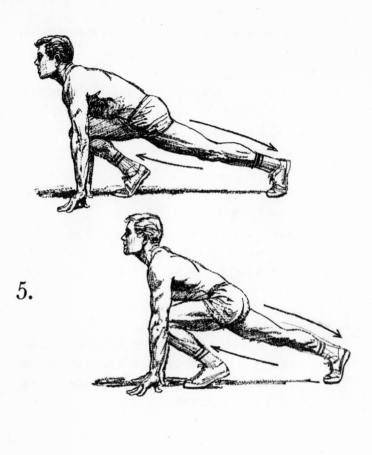

5.

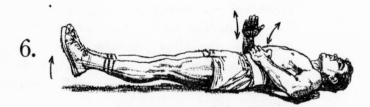

6.

5. SPRINTING—2 minutes

Squat down, knees bent, hands on floor, fingers pointed ahead, with left leg extended to rear. In one bouncing movement, reverse leg positions, bringing left foot up to hands, extending right leg to rear. Count one for each bounce. Repeat as often as you can for two minutes.

6. SUSTAINED LEG RAISE—2 minutes

Lie on your back, raise both legs 4 to 5 inches off the floor. Hold them there as long as possible, for the full two minutes if you can. At the same time, slap abdomen vigorously, first with one hand, then with the other, while breathing as deeply as you can.

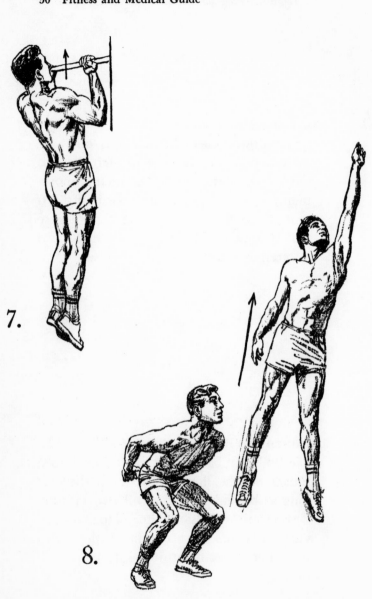

7.

8.

7. CHINNING—1 minute
    Chin yourself repeatedly. You can buy a
    bar, or improvise one, to set up across a
    doorway.

8. JUMP UP—1 minute
    Stand near a wall, bend knees, bring hands
    behind back, and position yourself for a
    leap upward. Jump, and keep jumping,
    always trying to come within one inch of
    your highest point. Repeat as often as pos-
    sible in the one-minute period.

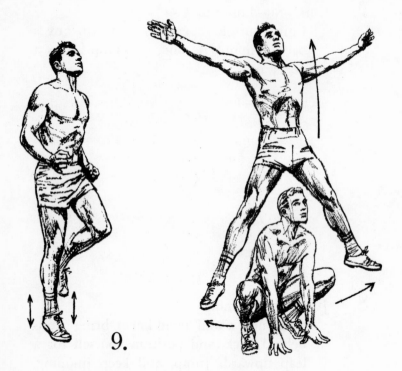

9.

9. MODIFIED STATIONARY RUN—6 minutes

Run in place, raising each foot at least 4 inches off floor. Each time right foot hits floor count 1. After 100 counts, do 10 spread jumps as illustrated. Repeat running and jumping for 6 minutes.

The spread jump: With feet together, sit down on heels, fingertips touching floor in front. Jump up; in mid-air, raise hands to shoulder level or slightly above and, at the same time, spread the feet as far apart as you can. Return to sit-on-heels position.

PHASE THREE

If you've been walking as your phase three activity and wish to continue doing so, increase the distance to two miles. And progressively cut down on the time—by walking faster and by alternating brief bursts of running with the walking.

If you prefer some other activity instead of or as an occasional alternative to walking, increase the effort. Make your jogging more vigorous. Or if you're swimming, you can try to swim 100 yards, breathe deeply for a minute, then swim another 100 yards. Keep repeating, gradually increasing repetitions and speed.

PROGRESSION RECORD

EXERCISE	5th week	6th week	7th week	8th week
1				
2				
3				
4				
5				
6				
7				
8				
9				
2-mile time				

THIRD MONTH

If your workouts have gone well in the second month, showing definite progression, and if you're entirely comfortable with the exercises, you're ready to go to a still higher level.

PHASE ONE— *The Warm-Up*

These exercises remain the same. You can continue them exactly as before (pages 22–24), or it may be possible now for you to reduce the time or repetitions for each one by about one-half.

PHASE TWO

To make this part of your workout more challenging and rewarding, some of the exercises have been modified to make them more strenuous, other have been lengthened. Your Phase Two activities will now take just a few minutes longer but they will be minutes well spent.

As the exercises become more difficult and as you master them and do them for longer periods and gradually increase the pace of doing them—and also are able to go from one to the next more rapidly so that the workout becomes almost continuous—you increase not only the strength and endurance of the muscles but of the whole body system.

Again, because it is so important, this cautionary note: Don't go overboard. Take it easy at the outset. Try to step up the pace a little in each successive workout. If at any time you feel you've overdone—as indicated by failure to recover quickly after a workout, long continued breathlessness, fatigue next day—drop the pace well back for the next workout and thereafter increase it less rapidly.

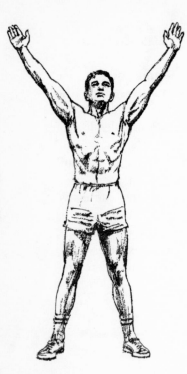

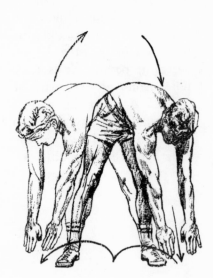

1.

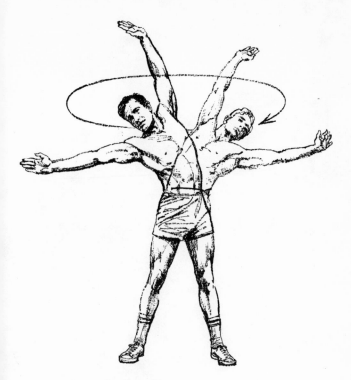

Third Month, Phase Two

1. BENDS—3 minutes
    Stand erect, feet 18 to 24 inches apart,
    hands overhead. Keeping knees straight,
    bend forward and down to touch the floor
    with fingers of both hands—first, outside
    the left foot, then between the feet, finally
    outside the right foot. Return to upright
    position. Then, with hands stretched over-
    head, bend the upper part of the body
    around in as big a circle as you can. Repeat
    for 3 minutes, as many times as you can.

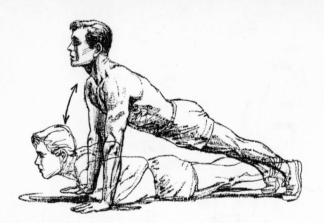

2.

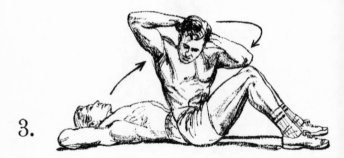

3.

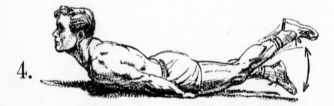

4.

2.   PUSHUPS—3 minutes
Do full-length pushups. Start with chest on floor, hands directly under shoulders, back and legs straight. Repeat as many times as possible in 3 minutes.

3.   FURTHER MODIFIED SITUPS—2 minutes
Lie on your back, arms clasped behind the head. Sit up and raise legs, with knees bent, twisting so you can touch your left elbow to right knee. Return to starting position. Repeat, this time touching right elbow to left knee. Keep repeating as often as possible in 2 minutes, alternating direction of twist each time.

4.   FLUTTER KICK—3 minutes
Lie on stomach, hands under thighs. Arch back to bring chest and head up. Flutter kick. Keep legs 8 to 10 inches apart; move them from hip with slight bend in knees. Count each kick as one.

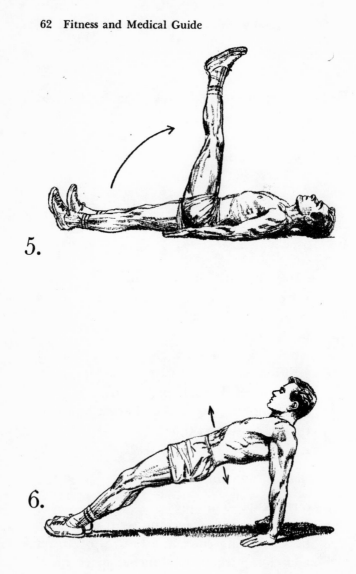

5.

6.

5.   LEG RAISE AND LOWER—no time period
Lying on your back, legs together and knees stiff, raise both legs to vertical position—then *slowly* lower them to floor. Repeat 20 times.

6.   GUT WHIPPER—2 minutes
Position yourself, back toward floor, with hands and heels supporting the body. Swing your middle up and down rapidly —as high up as you can make it go. Continue for 2 minutes.

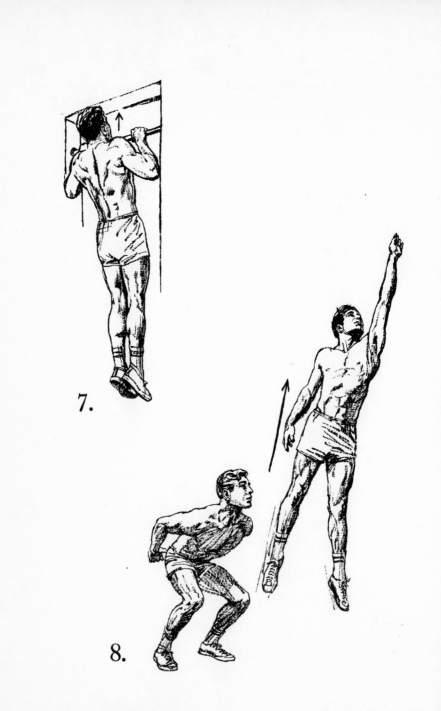

7.

8.

7. CHINNING—no time period

With palms forward—a position that helps more to add arm and back muscle strength —chin yourself, getting the chin well above the bar, extending the arms fully upon return. Repeat as many times as you can.

8. JUMP UP—2 minutes

Stand near a wall, bend knees, bring hands behind back, and position yourself for an upward leap. Jump, and keep jumping, always trying to come within an inch of your highest mark. Repeat as often as possible in 2 minutes.

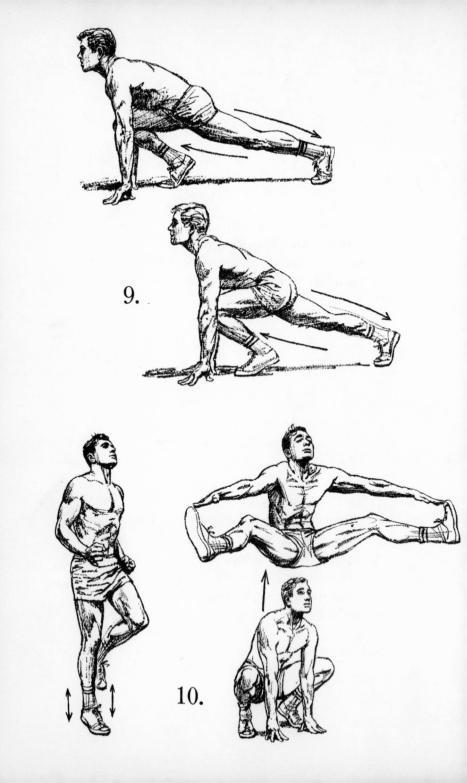

9.

10.

9. SPRINTING—3 minutes

Squat, knees bent, hands on floor, fingers pointed ahead, left leg extended to rear. In one bouncing movement, reverse leg positions, bringing left foot up to hands, extending right to rear. Count one for each bounce. Repeat as often as you can in 3 minutes.

10. FURTHER MODIFIED STATIONARY RUN— 6 minutes

Run in place, raising each foot at least 4 inches off floor. Each time right foot hits floor count 1. After 100 counts, do 10 toe-touch jumps as illustrated. Repeat running and jumping for 6 minutes.

Toe touch jumps: Sit on heels, fingertips touching the floor. Jump up, spread legs to side and raise them as high as you can, keeping the feet straight, and touch toes with fingertips in mid-air.

NOTE: If you are unable to do toe touch jumps, continue with spread jump used during second month but increase gradually to 20 jumps for every 100 counts.

PHASE THREE

Keep on with the activity you prefer and have used in preceding months—and progressively make it more vigorous. For example, you can work up to this: walk a mile, run half a mile, walk a quarter mile, sprint 200 yards, then walk another mile. Or you can use other variations to cover about a 3-mile distance as briskly as possible.

PROGRESSION RECORD

EXERCISE	9th week	10th week	11th week	12th week
1				
2				
3				
4				
5				
6				
7				
8				
9				
10				

3-mile time

After Three Months

Some men reach a very high level of fitness in three months—as high as they can or wish to go. Others need six months or even more to get into peak shape.

If you feel you'd like to further enhance your strength and endurance, you can do so by continuing with the third month workouts, progressively increasing their strenuousness by increasing repetitions in given time periods and then by extending the time periods a bit.

If you feel you have reached the level you want to be at, you can maintain it by continuing your workouts at the same pace. For maintenance purposes, it may be possible to do well with three workouts a week—although five may well be preferable.

No question—an hour a day is a lot of time. But it's an hour, you probably have decided by this time, well spent when it's devoted to making and keeping you vigorous, better able to get your daily job done without undue fatigue and with energy left over; and, as you may have had occasion by this time to discover, better able to get full enjoyment out of your hunting, fishing or other outdoor recreational activities.

There is no substitute—no pill, potion or anything else—for invigorating exercise.

You can add to your basic workout program or make some substitutions. There is room for flexibility.

Isometrics, for example, can be added; they need take little extra time. If you like to work with weights, you can use weight training—perhaps once or twice a week in place of the Phase Two activities of the basic program.

4 Try Jogging

If you should happen to be around the University of Florida track some morning between 6:45 and 7:30, you may see a group of men, young and middle-aged, enthusiastically working up steam by walking briskly, breaking into a trot, walking again, then trotting some more.

Similarly, at the University of Oregon track, early in the morning, late in the afternoon, and at various times of day, you'll often find men, many of them professors and university staff members, jogging around individually and in groups in the effort to build and maintain fitness, and evidently having fun in the process.

Late in the afternoon in some YMCA gyms, you can find men who stop in after work to go jogging around above the basketball court on the 20- to 25-laps-to-the-mile tracks, some of them covering as much as 1,000 miles a year.

Jogging through parks, on semi-secluded tracks of high schools, even on some golf course fairways—early morning, afternoon, evening, almost anytime—is becoming increasingly popular.

And for good reasons.

Values of Jogging

Jogging, say its advocates, many of them physicians, is a simple, practical aid in developing both muscular

70

strength and general endurance. It's inexpensive and requires no special skill. Anybody can do it—and get a lot out of it.

Says Dr. Warren R. Guild of Harvard, an authority on sports medicine and fitness: "This quicker method of covering the ground can cram a more extensive workout into a shorter period of time . . . For a man 35 years old to take up the 100 yard dash would be ridiculous, but for this same man to jog along comfortably for longer and longer distances is quite a different matter."

Says Dr. Sid Robinson of Indiana University: "For the benefit you get out of it, running probably requires less time than any other activity. Walking is good but still is too time consuming if you do enough of it. Golf takes you too long to play. Running is one sport that requires no equipment—nor partners. You can just go out and do it. You don't need a lifeguard. And a handball court, or a tennis court, or a squash racket are not necessary."

University of Oregon track Coach Bill Bowerman, who is credited with doing much to popularize jogging in this country, picked up the idea on a visit to New Zealand where he saw men of all ages jogging all over the island—on tracks, out in the hills, down country roads, through city streets.

Bowerman, 52 and a 205-pounder in pretty fair shape, spent a month in New Zealand and started running with the Auckland Joggers Club, working his distance up to two to three miles a day. He lost no weight but knocked 3 inches off his 38-inch waist in the month, continued the jogging when he got home, dropped his weight gradually to 185. Before long he was organizing joggers clubs around the University in Eugene and then in other Oregon communities—"No dues, no membership, no minutes, just jog."

Obviously, not everybody can be expected to like jogging. But many men do—including some well-known ones.

George Romney, Michigan governor, gets up at 5 in the morning and starts his day with a one to two-mile jog. John Glenn gets out and runs. So does TV actor Richard Chamberlain. Dr. Dwight J. Ingle, chairman of the University of Chicago's Department of Physiology, is out six days a week, usually knocking off about two miles. Ingle has run up to six miles but considers that too far for him at the age of 56, prefers to go "just far enough to get comfortably fatigued."

There is evidence of the value of running for knocking down blood cholesterol levels. A study of 156 marathon runners ranging from 17 to 63 years of age showed their average cholesterol level to be much lower than that for the general public.

Other studies carried out at Kent State University in Ohio with middle-aged men have shown that running—coupled with other exercises—produces a substantial decrease in blood fat levels.

Particularly for the outdoorsman, jogging makes good sense—if you like or can learn to like it.

You can use jogging as an alternative to walking for your phase three activities under the progressive fitness program. It's good exercise for virtually all muscles and certainly for leg muscles you make use of in the field. It stimulates circulation, gives you more wind.

You can jog by yourself—or find a willing companion.

You may even have no great difficulty in getting together a small group and organizing a little joggers club
of your own. (If you interest others, it's a good idea to
urge them first to get a medical check and an O.K. from
their physicians. It might not be a bad idea at all to urge
them at the same time to couple their jogging with the
progressive fitness program.)

How to Do It

Take it easy at the beginning. Start with a jog that is
only a little faster than a brisk walk. Jog until you begin
to puff. Then walk. Then jog again.

Your body should be upright—not bent forward.
Keep the buttocks in, not protruding; the back straight,
not arched. Bend the elbows. Breathe through nose and
mouth.

The objective is to start at a comfortable level and
make progress by gradually exerting yourself more and
more. At the beginning, you can jog for fifty yards, walk
for fifty yards, keep alternating, and cover about a mile.
As you keep working out, you'll find yourself able to
increase the distance, to jog more and walk less, and to
jog faster, even interspersing some sprints, running as
fast as you can for fifty yards, then dropping back to a
jog or walk. Over a period of several months, possibly
less, you may find it possible to progress until you can
cover as much as three miles at a good pace, walking
very little of the time.

You can clock yourself, but there is no need to set any
specific time goals. People differ considerably. Some can
run for a year and still not be able to do a mile in under

8 minutes, or even run continuously for a mile without knocking themselves out.

Your aim isn't to set any records, only to gradually push up your energy expenditure and, in doing so, your wind, strength and endurance. Even if you never get to the point of running hard for a mile, you can expect to get a lot of good out of jogging.

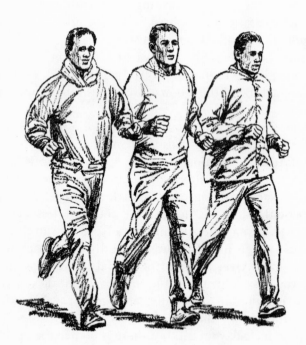

5 What You Can Do with Isometrics

It sounds too good to be true. It is.

For some years now, a muscle-building system called isometrics has been enjoying a spectacular vogue. Newspapers, books, magazines, even phonograph records have trumpeted the virtues of isometrics and propagandized, often innocently but nevertheless mistakenly: "No sweat. A minute a day and you can be in top shape."

Isometrics involve muscular contractions without movement. The system is based on the old overload principle which holds that when a muscle is required to perform work beyond the usual intensity it will respond with growth. In the system, one set of muscles may be pitted against another—or against an immovable object such as a doorway, floor or chair.

As popularly practiced, a muscle is worked out for six seconds once a day—no repetitions. And that, it has been claimed, is enough to double strength in as little as twenty weeks.

There's no question but that isometrics can be useful, but the whole subject has been grossly oversimplified. Isometrics can supplement but not completely replace isotonic exercises such as pushups, situps, etc. To be physically fit in general—and certainly to be in top form for hunting and other outdoor activities—you need muscular strength PLUS.

Strength is the ability to work against a specified resistance. Additionally, you need:

1. Muscular endurance—which is the ability of a muscle to respond repetitively for a relatively long period of time.

2. Flexibility or muscular elasticity so you can use the muscle effectively throughout its whole range of motion.

3. Cardiovascular-pulmonary efficiency—the adaptive response of heart, blood vessels and lungs to work and exercise.

Isometrics can help develop muscular strength. But for the other needs, you have to get down on the floor and do pushups and situps and other isotonic exercises; you have to work the muscles through their whole range; you have to work them repeatedly; and you have to sweat at the job and give the heart and blood vessels and lungs a workout. There is no shortcut.

Other Facts About Isometrics

Is it true that isometrics can double muscle strength in twenty weeks—which means a 5 percent gain per week? A more realistic figure, experts have been finding recently, may be 2 percent a week—and even that, some suggest, may be generous.

What may be another misconception is the idea that one contraction a day is all that is needed for maximum daily gain. Recent experiments seem to contradict this. Says Dr. Arthur H. Steinhaus of George Williams College, one of the most respected authorities in the field of physiology: "You can't get maximum growth. with just one contraction a day. It has to be five to ten contractions."

Still another misconception is that isometric exercises are easy, virtually effortless. On the contrary, if done properly, they can produce as much sweat as isotonics. To get maximum strength-building value out of them, you have to progress to the point of maximum or near-maximum contraction.

Finally, there is this to be considered. Isometrics are specific exercises. You work out a single muscle area at a time. If you were to depend upon isometrics alone to work out all the muscles you need to tone up to get into good shape, you would probably find them at least as time-consuming and dull as isotonics.

Where Isometrics Fit In

You're better off making the progressive fitness program (Chapter 3) the basis for getting and staying in shape, using isometrics, if you wish, to supplement that program.

The isometric exercises that follow are useful for further development of specific major muscles and muscle areas. You may wish to use all or to pick out a few to help add strength where you feel you need it most.

There is no special order to be followed. Nor need you do all—or the series you choose—at one time. You can, if you like, do a few in the morning, others at various times during the day.

Do little breathing during a contraction; breathe deeply between contractions.

Maintain each contraction no more than eight seconds. And for the first week or two, exert only about 50 percent of what you believe is the maximum force you're capable of exerting. Thereafter, gradually increase the force. As you go along, you can begin to repeat the contractions several times a day.

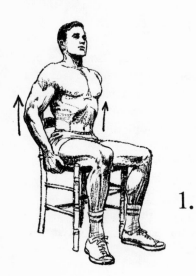

1.

2.

1.   PULL-UP (for arms and shoulders)
       Sitting straight, with shoulders back,
       tightly grip sides of chair with both hands.
       Pull up hard.

2.   LIFT-UP (for shoulders, arms, abdomen)
       While seated, grip sides of chair with both
       hands. Hold the legs straight out. With
       back kept straight, lean forward until
       you're in position to try to lift your whole
       body about one inch off the chair.

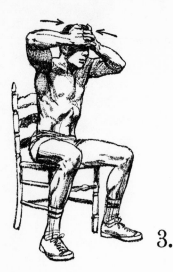

3.

4.

5.

3.   HAND PRESS (for shoulders, arms, chest)
      Sit up straight, shoulders back, chest out,
      arms in front of chest. Put one fist inside
      the other and, using full strength of your
      arms and shoulders, press together.

4.   BACK PULL-UP (to strengthen back muscles)
      With back kept as straight as possible, lean
      forward in chair. Grasp both legs above
      ankles and bring them back into position
      that allows you to pull straight up using
      only your back muscles.

5.   LEG HOLD (for leg muscles)
      Seated in chair, cross left ankle over right.
      Rest feet on floor, with legs bent at 90
      degree angle. Push up forcibly with right
      leg, trying to straighten it, while resisting
      just as forcibly with left leg. REPEAT
      with legs reversed.

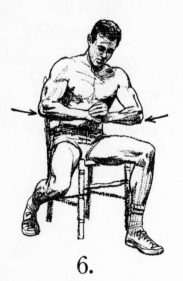

6.

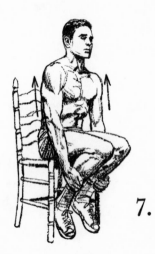

7.

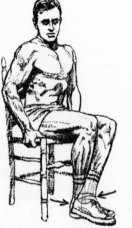

8.

6. HEAD PUSH, FORWARD (for neck muscles)
Either seated or standing, interlace fingers of hands, place against forehead—and, while resisting with the hands, try to push head forward.

7. HEAD PUSH, BACK (for neck muscles)
Place interlaced fingers of hands behind the head—and, while pulling forward hard with the hands, try equally hard to push the head back.

8. HEAD PUSH, SIDE (for neck muscles)
Place palm of left hand against left side of head—and, while resisting hard with the hand, try to move head to the left. REPEAT with right hand on right side.

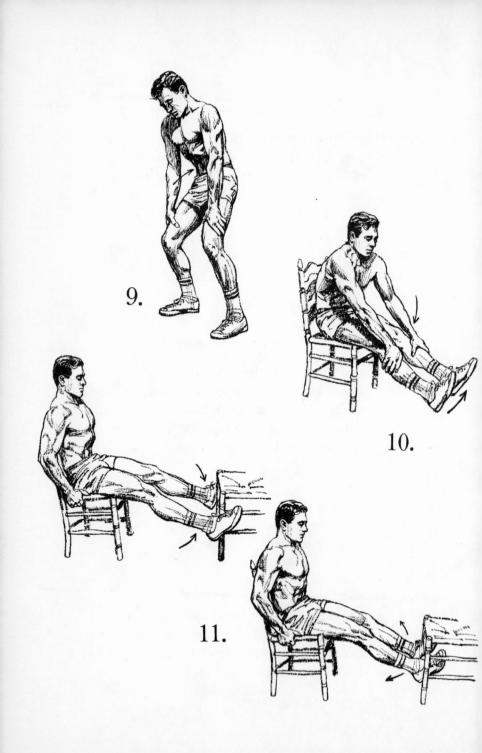

9.

10.

11.

9. GUT TIGHTENER (to tone abdominal muscles)
    Stand with knees slightly bent, upper part
    of body leaning slightly forward, hands
    resting on knees. Pull in gut, contracting
    abdominal muscles hard.

10. GUT TIGHTENER #2
    Sitting with legs held straight out, bend
    forward, grasp legs just below the knees.
    Push down with the hands while simul-
    taneously pressing up with the legs.

11. LEG-CHAIR PRESS AND PULL (for inner and
    outer thigh muscles)
    Sit in one chair, extend the legs, place
    ankles outside front legs of a sturdy second
    chair. Keeping legs extended, try forcibly
    to bring them together against opposition
    of the chair. REPEAT with ankles inside
    chair legs, exerting pressure outward.

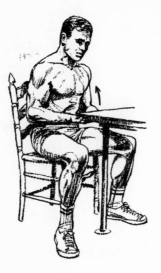

12.

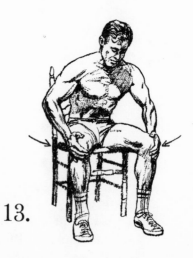

13.

12. TABLE RAISER (for upper arm muscles)
Sitting erect, place hands, palms up, under heavy table or desk, with forearms parallel to top surface of table or desk. Push up, trying to lift.

13. KNEE HOLD (for shoulder, forearm and hip muscles)
While seated, lean forward and grasp outsides of knees. Exert spreading pressure with knees while resisting with hands.

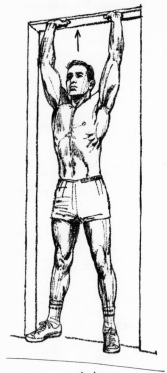

14.

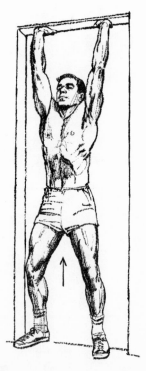

15.

14. DOOR FRAME PUSH (for arm and trunk muscles)

Standing in doorway, place hands against door frame and push upward, with knees locked.

15. DOOR FRAME PUSH #2 (for thigh muscles)

Stand in doorway—this time with knees bent and elbows locked. Press upward with the force coming from the thighs.

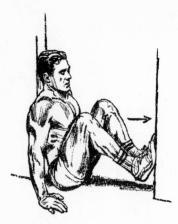

16.

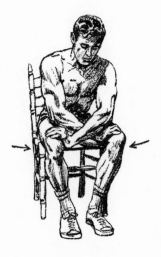

17.

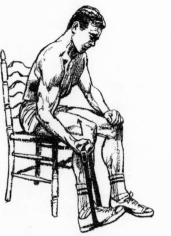

18.

16. DOOR FRAME PUSH #3 (for hips and thighs)
Sit in the doorway—with back against one
side and feet against opposite side, legs
bent. Exert pressure you can feel in the
thighs and hips.

17. CRISSCROSS PRESS (for legs and chest)
Seated on edge of chair, with feet on floor
about 4 inches apart, lean forward and
place left hand against inside of right knee,
right hand against inside of opposite knee.
Try to bring knees together while simul-
taneously holding them apart with the
hands.

18. BELT PULL (for the biceps)
Use your trouser belt. Fasten buckle. Sit
down and place closed loop of belt under
arch of right shoe. Grasp belt with right
hand and exert pressure you feel in biceps.
REPEAT on opposite side.

6   Special Occasion Workouts

The progressive fitness program can be counted on to toughen you up and get you into good shape for any and all outdoor activities. If you're planning something special—perhaps some rugged mountain climbing or a ski vacation, for example—you may want to tack on a few special exercises in preparation. Leg muscles, of course, come in for particularly heavy stress in skiing and climbing.

Walking about on tip-toe whenever you get the chance is one good—and simple—strengthener for lower leg muscles.

As an extra aid in toughening up thigh muscles, you can sit on the edge of a table, lift your legs, lower them, keep repeating. Then add weights and lift. You don't have to go out and buy weights for this purpose; you can use some heavy workshop items, even canned goods, stuffed into a pillow case. Work up to lifting 35 pounds or more with each leg.

Another good leg strengthener: While shaving, stand on one leg and flex the knee. Repeat with the other leg.

Beware of deep knee bends. They've often been advocated for skiers—and, in fact, for many other sports participants. But deep bends—and also the "duck waddle," another traditional leg strengthener—are now generally disapproved by medical authorities. Both exercises may lead to serious injury to the internal and supporting structures of the knee joint, one of the most vulnerable parts of the body.

In the deep knee bend, you move from standing position to full squat. In the duck waddle, you get into a full squat and then travel. "Both exercises," the American Medical Association has warned, "involve complete flexion and often twisting of the knee which can result in cumulative deterioration or immediate injury to the meniscus (cushioning cartilage) of the joint." Instead of deep knee bends, you can use a few half knee bends now and then for leg strengthening.

Rope jumping is valuable for strengthening muscles in calves and thighs. And you don't even need a rope. Jump an inch or two off the floor and imagine you're using a rope.

Stair climbing can add extra toughening for your leg muscles. If you work or live in a building with an elevator, start by not using the elevator for the full distance—up or down (climbing down as well as up is good exercise). Start with a couple of floors of climbing and add on gradually. Note: Don't dash up steps; let the muscles of your legs push you up.

If you can get out into the country and find a hillside —and the rougher the terrain, the better—practice running up and down. That's good for your legs—and your wind.

Your wind, of course, is important in many activities. Especially at high altitudes with their rarefied atmosphere, having plenty of lung power and high circulatory efficiency is a big help in minimizing lethargy and fatigue.

If you're following the progressive fitness program, you're undoubtedly experiencing considerable improvement in wind. If you're planning a high-altitude trip, you might want to try a bit harder for several weeks before you go off to increase the tempo of the exercises, do more walking or jogging and at a faster pace and over longer distances to buck up your lung and circulatory efficiency still more.

7 If Time Is Short—
a One-Month Workup

The best way to work up to a high level of physical fitness—to get into top trim so you can have more fun out of every hunting and fishing trip or other outdoor recreational activity—is to use a program such as the one in Chapter 3 which progressively increases your strength and endurance over a period of time.

But suppose you're starting from scratch and have little time—a trip all planned and set and coming up fast. You'd like before then—in the next month—to get into as good shape as you possibly can.

That's what this special program is designed to help you do. It's no substitute, over the long run, for the full fitness program. But if your doctor checks you out as basically healthy and able to undertake it, you can expect it to bring about an impressive improvement within a month. In fact, the results, though short of ideal, are likely to be impressive enough to encourage you, once you're back from your trip, to go to work on the full program.

How to Use the One-Month Program

There are just six special exercises. They should be used in conjunction with the warm-up exercises described in Chapter 3. Start with the warm-ups, then do all six of the special exercises in the order shown.

Work out three times in the first week—on alternate days. Add a fourth workout the second week. For the final two weeks, exercise at least five times a week.

Start off with a comfortable number of repetitions for each exercise—say fifteen times.

Gradually, from workout to workout, increase the number of repetitions. To get into the best possible shape, you have to increase the demand on the body. But curb any overenthusiasm. Don't try to go all-out immediately; you'll get stiff and sore and actually delay progress if you do.

In the early workouts, don't hesitate to pause between exercises if you feel that necessary. Stop, take some long, deep breaths, then go on.

As you go along in successive workouts, try to reach the point where you're spending half an hour or more on the six exercises and the workout is almost continuous, without pauses between exercises.

You can make the exercise bar yourself. The one shown is made from 1¼-inch black pipe, 48 inches long, with handholds of rubberized friction tape wound 12–16 inches from each end.

Follow the suggestions in Chapter 3 for tapering and cooling off after your workouts.

And use a Phase Three activity (see explanation in Chapter 3). For the first week, get out at least three times and walk a mile each time. You can do this on the days you use the special exercises or on the other days. Don't make the pace exhausting.

In the second week, get in at least four walks of a mile each, gradually stepping up the pace.

In the final two weeks, increase your walking distance to two miles and make the pace as brisk as possible. Try to work in some jogging, alternating it with walking, over the two-mile distance.

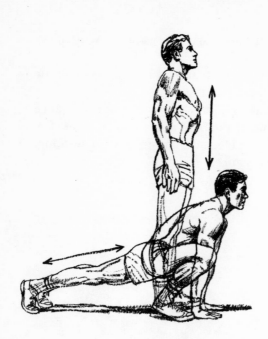

1.

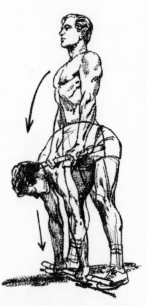

2.

1. DOWN AND OUT (for legs, arms, shoulders, general toning)

Stand erect, feet about 12 inches apart. Squat and place hands on floor between feet. Thrust legs backward as far as possible, straightening the body—then jump feet back to hands in squat position and stand erect again.

2. BACK STRENGTH

Stand erect with feet apart. Grasp exercise pipe palms down. Touch pipe to toes, keeping knees locked. Straighten up to starting position.

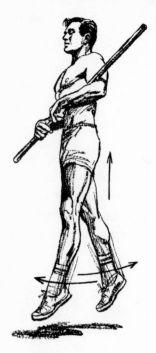

3.

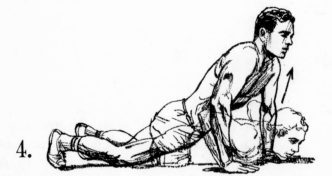

4.

3. WIND PLUS

Stand erect with right foot about 2 feet in front of left. Jump both feet off floor, switching them in mid-air, and land with left foot about 2 feet in front of right. Then jump back to starting position.

Each time you repeat the exercise, hold the exercise pipe like a gun—in a different carrying position: on one shoulder, then the other; in the crook of one arm, then the other; cradled in both arms.

4. CRAWL POWER

Lie face down on floor. Place hands flat on floor by shoulders. Push up, keeping feet and knees on floor. Lower chest to floor again.

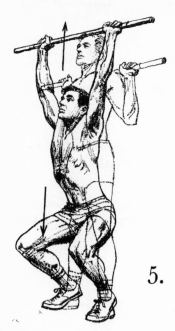

5.

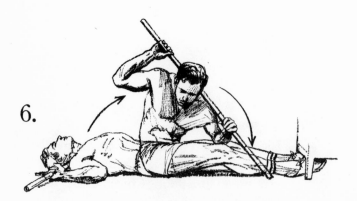

6.

5. LEG, CHEST AND SHOULDER STRENGTH

Stand erect. Hold exercise pipe behind neck, across shoulders, chest expanded, arm muscles taut. Lower body by bending knees about half way down—and, at the same time, push bar vigorously up over head. Straighten knees, bring bar down across shoulders.

6. GUT HARDENER

Sit on floor, legs together, knees straight, feet hooked under heavy chair or other solid object. Hold exercise pipe behind neck, across shoulders. Lie down with back on floor. Sit up and twist to right, touching left end of pipe to floor outside right leg. Lie back down on floor. Sit up again and twist to left, touching right end of pipe to floor outside left leg.

8   Some Special Notes

Drugs and Other Fads

Recently an American Medical Association Committee on Medical Aspects of Sports found it necessary to put it on the line: Any athlete or sportsman "who experiments with pep pills, whiffs of oxygen, odd dietary supplements and other such fads in the hope of improving performance is doomed to disappointment and may even be courting bodily harm."

With their premium on endurance and top performance, sports always have been fertile soil for experimentation with "ergogenic aids," so-called because they're supposed to increase stamina.

But the faddish use of such aids, the Committee says, is of no more value for sports success than the superstition of never changing underwear during a winning streak—and may even be downright hazardous.

The Hormone Hazard

One of the new and dangerous fads involves use of androgenic-anabolic steroids—drugs chemically similar to the nautral male hormone, testosterone. They were originally developed to put weight on debilitated older people, retard bone deterioration sometimes associated with old age, and relieve some forms of anemia—always under close medical supervision.

Somehow—nobody knows exactly when—a few body-conscious specimens who like to show off their muscles on Southern California beaches started the fad of taking the steroid pills to try to bulge up their physiques some more and improve their stamina. Apparently, many healthy young athletes across the country soon took up the fad and it's suspected some full-grown sportsmen may have become its victims.

Do the pills do any good? Hardly.

When University of California at Los Angeles investigators recently gave a series of strength tests to men taking the steroids, they found that the medication produced no improvement at all. Moreover, some of the men began to complain of dizziness and muscle aches.

Other investigators warn that men taking the steroids for long periods risk decreased libido and shrinking of the testicles since the drugs tend to reduce the body's production of natural testosterone. Unfortunately, the scientists note, such effects are "insidious, not immediately apparent."

Pep Pills

Airmen in World War II sometimes were given pep pills—amphetamines—to keep them alert on long, dangerous missions. When Astronaut Gordon Cooper's automatic controls failed, he was ordered to take an amphetamine so his reflexes would be sharp for manual reentry.

But if pep pills—also known as "goof balls"—can be of some help when medically prescribed for special situations, their indiscriminate use can be dangerous.

The drugs can't prevent fatigue; they obscure it. They stimulate the central nervous system. A pill-taker feels the stimulation and has a false sense of invigoration. But a feeling of restlessness, tenseness, even sleeplessness, may develop.

There is a particular danger, too, in the let down which most people experience as the drug wears off. It often comes without warning, may bring with it overpowering fatigue which can be dangerous in a driving situation or in many others. There are other hazards—of habituation and overdosage. When the stimulating effect of a pill wears off, there is temptation to repeat the dose and often larger doses are needed.

Repeated use of pep pills can lead to trouble not only in sleeping but even in standing and sitting still. The eyes of abusers often become dilated, the breath gets bad; they may go on fighting fatigue for hours or days but end up collapsing.

It's also a fact that excessive dosage with amphetamines may lead to elevated blood pressure, irritability, abdominal distress, chest pains and rapid heart rate.

Healthy endurance doesn't come in the shape of pills. It's obtainable only by improving physical equipment, building up natural reserves of energy that can take care of strenuous activities and even emergencies no pill can handle.

Fatigue—Normal and Abnormal

Muscles, of course, are subject to exhaustion. Yet they can bounce back fast—even after a stiff workout. Using an instrument, the ergometer, to measure contractions in volunteers lifting weights, investigators have found that after twenty minutes of strenuous activity muscles may lose half or more of their power—but, after twelve minutes of rest, they recover as much as 90 percent and even more of peak force. With each repetition of exhausting work, the exhaustion of course tends to set in a little earlier.

People vary greatly in fatigue resistance—and a prime reason is physical condition. The importance of condition is obvious in the performance of trained athletes. But not long ago, investigators from one university set up shop at a fairgrounds and got sixty passing men, ranging in age from 19 to 61, to step up and take a test ride on an ergometer-equipped bicycle.

There were no trained athletes in the group. Virtually all the men were at least a little flabby and a few pounds overweight. Yet those taking some kind of moderate regular exercise—light calisthenics or just a periodic dip in a backyard or Y pool—turned out to have on the average 20 percent greater working capacity.

As already noted, regular exercise does much more than increase muscle size. It conditions the heart to pump blood more efficiently—a greater volume with each beat. It conditions the lungs as well to function more effectively. And it increases circulation efficiency, opening up tiny blood vessels that extend into the muscles, improving both muscle nourishment and the process of getting rid of the by-products of activity. All of these are major factors in increasing strength, endurance and fatigue resistance.

With even light but regular exercise of almost any kind shown to be capable of increasing work capacity by

20 percent, you can expect a considerably greater increase in strength and endurance as you get yourself into shape with a progressive fitness program.

There is, of course, abnormal fatigue. Many physical disturbances can be responsible. If, for example, the thyroid, a little gland in the throat that paces energy-conversion processes, works under par, fatigue is a result. Diabetics who don't take enough insulin become fatigued because certain wastes pile up; on the other hand, if they take too much, they become fatigued because excess insulin removes too much blood sugar. A medical check-up can disclose physical problems behind abnormal fatigue and lead to their correction.

Tension is a common cause of abnormal fatigue. All of us are subject to tension; it's almost impossible to avoid. It's built up by job pressures, family problems, traffic, noise, crisis piled upon crisis in the news. It's tension, of course, which accounts for the mammoth sales of tranquilizers. In extreme cases, such drugs have their values. But most good physicians believe strongly that they should not be used except in extreme cases. They're potent drugs, not without their dangers.

"To use tranquilizers to relieve everyday stress and strain and conflict is to use a sledgehammer on a thumb tack," says Dr. Harry J. Johnson, President of Life Extension Foundation.

"Relaxation," he adds, "in small and large doses is the antidote to excessive tension. This does not mean rest—it means a change of activity. The best cure for tension fatigue is exercise."

Out of recent research come insights into the importance of the nervous system in fatigue. You've probably

had the experience of feeling bushed and then, moti-
vated by some unexpected pleasure or a sudden emergency, you found yourself able to summon instant
energy and get moving with an alacrity you would have
thought impossible a few minutes before.

The sensation of fatigue appears to reside in the
thalamus and hypothalamus areas of the brain. It also
appears to be countered by stimulation from another
brain area, the reticular formation. The latter acts in
response to messages coming through the nervous system
and it becomes less responsive—apparently the whole
nervous system does—when messages are monotonous.

Boredom, experts report, is one of the chief reasons
for fatigue experienced by industrial and office workers.

As one leading authority, Dr. Peter Karpovich of
Springfield College, has put it: "It is the nervous system
that gets tired first. When work is not interesting one
may tire sooner than with work that is harder but more
stimulating. This type of fatigue is really boredom although you may feel physically tired."

And it has been shown in such situations, Karpovich
says, that even a short break—it doesn't matter whether
for coffee, a snack or just a chat—is a big help.

Another insight comes from scientists who have been
investigating psychological barriers that interfere with
strength and endurance. Most of us, it seems clear, have
far more strength and energy than we normally use or
believe we have.

The Psychology of Stamina

Dr. Arthur E. Steinhaus ran a series of experiments at
George Williams College in Chicago. He put subjects to

work contracting their right arms isometrically. They were supposed to exert maximum force once a minute for thirty minutes—and instruments measured the force they exerted.

The tests were repeated after the subjects were given amphetamine—and also when a 22-caliber starter's gun was fired unexpectedly behind them to startle them into greater effort. And hypnosis was tried: subjects were told they were getting stronger.

Steinhaus found that amphetamine produced an average increase in force of 9.5 pounds. Even the gunshot led to a 4.5 pound increase. Best of all was simple suggestion under hypnosis; that upped the force by 18.3 pounds.

Not long ago, Dr. Stewart G. Wolf of the University of Oklahoma School of Medicine reported that most people "unconsciously and automatically limit their exertional efforts anywhere in the neighborhood of 50 percent of their capacity." He told of one study in which subjects were asked to hold weights in their extended arms as long as they could. After a rest period, they were given dummy pills which they thought contained a powerful antifatigue preparation. "This," says Wolf, "resulted in nearly doubling the endurance of the group."

Among the classic experiments in fatigue is the one by Dr. Arthur Bliss of the University of Cincinati in which a frail coed and a husky football player were asked to stand as long as they could with arms outstretched. The football man dropped his after ten minutes; he'd been told beforehand that, though it seemed easy, this was a tough test of stamina. The coed went right on holding out her arms without strain; she had been told that, though the task seemed hard, it really was easy.

Actually, says Bliss, "most of the suggestions that make you feel peppy or tired come from within. By weeding out negative ideas you can work and play harder."

Sleep

You need proper rest to get and keep in top shape. Generally, people need seven to eight hours of sleep but there is no standard requirement. There are people who can get by well on less, as little as six hours; others need more—as much as nine and ten hours.

It used to be thought that as people grow older, they can do with less sleep than in childhood and young adulthood. But recent research has upset the idea, indicating that older people may need just as much sleep as younger—and that some of the slowing down with age and the vague complaints of the elderly and even the middle-aged may be traceable simply to insufficient sleep.

It also used to be thought that there were some people who could get by with no more than four hours sleep—but modern research also tends to discount that. It has been established, for example, that even Thomas Edison, who claimed to sleep no more than three or fours hours a night, had a bed in his laboratory which he used during the day—and he didn't count those hours. About all that can be said with any certainty is that the right amount of sleep is an individual matter. You need

whatever amount—seven hours, nine hours, or something else—it takes to make you feel bright and in good
fettle next day.

The Insomnia Problem

Everybdy has it at times; it's a product of tension
and anxiety. Nobody has found a sure method of
putting every insomniac to sleep but some helpful insights into the problem have come out of recent research.

For one thing, it is impossible to stay awake indefin-
itely. Even the worst insomniac need not fear that he
will never sleep.

For another, it appears that if you lose sleep you can
catch up—and don't have to pay back as much as you've
lost. Studies have shown that volunteers in experiments,
after being deprived of sleep for as long as 100 hours
and then given a chance to sleep as long as they need to,
generally sleep no more than ten hours on the recovery
night. Then, for another three or four nights, they add
an extra hour or two. But the total amount of extra
sleep they feel the need for and actually take is a great
deal less than the amount lost.

(Incidentally, research has shown no evidence you
can put sleep "in the bank," storing it up by sleeping
extra for a couple of nights before a particularly difficult
period. On the contrary, there is evidence that it's of no
particular value, although taking a nap before you have
to stay up all night can be helpful.)

If you have any difficulty in falling asleep, the first
thing to do, if you possibly can, is to avoid worrying

about the difficulty. That compounds the problem. Worry increases the tension you went to bed with. That can mean tossing and turning all night, trying desperately to fall asleep and failing, until usually you drop off about 4 or 5 in the morning.

You drop off to sleep at that point because your body temperature, which goes through a daily cycle, varying as much as 2 degrees during the twenty-four hours, reaching a high in late afternoon or evening, reaches a low sometime between midnight and dawn, usually around 4 A.M. When temperature goes down, the body tends to relax more, you feel sleepiest, and sleep comes.

Sleep Aids

All of us make use of them—in the sense that we have a ritual about going to sleep. The ritual includes undressing, toilet and other preparations. For some people, it includes habitually eating or drinking something, relaxing with a book or other reading matter even if for no more than five or ten minutes. Such habitual activities are useful.

Recent research indicates it is important to prepare your room for sleeping by providing a comfortable temperature. "It seems important to have the bedroom cool and it's better to have the room cool enough so you require a blanket," reports Dr. Harold L. Williams, who directs sleep-research projects at Walter Reed Army Institute of Research in Washington, D.C.

Keeping a window open to get outside fresh air apparently has no basic importance. Some people sleep well with windows closed; others, Dr. Williams notes, find that if they don't open a window, they can't get to sleep because it's part of their habit pattern of getting to sleep.

Counting sheep has its value. In Russian medicine, sleep is used as a therapeutic tool (we've only begun to experiment with prolonged sleep as a treatment very recently). To get their patients to sleep and keep them asleep, Russian doctors have found that almost any rhythmic stimulation is useful. Regular, repeated, monotonous stimuli tend to induce sleep. Counting sheep provides such stimulation. So, too, does a loud-ticking bedroom clock.

Should sleeping pills be used? Certainly not indiscriminately. Their regular use can be hazardous. But some physicians believe a properly prescribed pill can be valuable when a man has somehow broken his sleeping pattern and is having trouble reestablishing it. A sleeping pill taken for two or three nights sometimes can help get the pattern going again.

Smoking and Drinking

It is not within the province of this book to review the arguments about the possible role of cigarette smoking in lung cancer or other health problems.

Just this practical note for the sportsman who smokes: For a time before you have to exert maximum effort in any activity, it is advisable to avoid smoking. The ability to produce maximum effort is related to capacity for taking in and ultilizing oxygen. Ten inhalations of cigarette smoke have been found to reduce the ability of the airways to pass oxygen along to the lungs by as much as 50 percent. The reduction—which comes about through muscle contraction and nervous reflex—lasts for as long as an hour.

As for alcohol, it has a sedative-tranquilizing action. Its value, in moderate amount, at the end of a stimulating or difficult day in producing relaxation is recognized by many. But it should not be used before or during any activity calling for energy, endurance or skill.

Unlike most foods, alcohol requires no digestion. It passes directly through the walls of the stomach and intestine into the blood stream and then to all organs of the body. When it reaches the brain, it produces a general dulling effect. For hours afterward, nerve-muscle coordination is impaired to some extent, enough to cause a marked loss of skill. Physical capacity, too, is lowered.

9   Nutrition and Diet

While it's possible to be well-nourished and not be fit, you can't be totally fit without being well-nourished.

There isn't—or shouldn't be—anything mysterious or complex about good nutrition. But that can be hard to believe if you're exposed even only occasionally to the seemingly endless array of new and often weird diets and diatribes in magazines, books and newspapers.

Analyze them and you find that generally they make either one or another of two claims:

1. That some specific foods are so vital they have to be eaten to the exclusion of others;

2. That certain specific combinations of foods are the panaceas for—the painless, effortless means for arriving at—good health.

Both claims are false.

And there are plenty of other misleading notions about nutrition we might as well dispose of before getting to the simple truth.

Fads and Fallacies

Writing not long ago in an American Medical Association publication, one physician and nutrition authority emphasized that "One of the paths to fitness is to select and consume a proper diet without frills, fads, fallacies, frauds, fears and furbelows."

And he proceeded to note just a few of the latter:

"We have, for example, the advocates of so-called natural foods, which in general means foods grown on soil fertilized with natural fertilizers rather than synthesized chemicals. We have those who would virtually discontinue the use of insecticides to guard against possible dangers, often very vague, of chemical poisoning. We have the advocates of all sorts of bizarre food fads, ranging from the idea that cooking in aluminum will predispose to cancer to the tradition that an apple a day will keep the doctor away."

Taking up the often-repeated idea that white bread is not worth eating because "all the nutritional value has been refined out of it," Dr. Harry Johnson of the Life Extension Foundation, a nonprofit organization devoted to health care, has remarked: "All bread is nutritionally good . . . It makes little difference whether it is whole wheat bread, rye or enriched white bread. A slice of each has essentially the same proteins and the same overall nutritional value . . . All of the common types of bread are equally well digested, but the white bread made from enriched, refined flour has some advantages over the others. It is usually better tolerated by those who have difficulty with their digestion."

And Dr. Johnson adds: "Some years ago we had the black-strap molasses and wheat-germ fad foisted on the public. More recently we had the vinegar and honey nonsense promoted with an air of authority. There is no food that has any special health value, nor any drink that has any special health benefit. All clean food is health food. Special grinding or mechanical mixing processes do not improve the nutritional value of food. The only thing that is special about these touted preparations is the price."

Do oysters, raw eggs, lean meat and olives increase a man's potency? Not on your life. They contribute to health and well-being but have no special potency effects.

This is just one of many still widely prevalent fallacious notions about diet which nutrition researchers are struggling to eliminate.

Here are some others:

• That fish and celery are brain foods. It's an idea that may have arisen because brain and nerve tissues are rich in phosphorus—and fish provides phosphorus-containing materials. But so do meat, poultry, eggs, milk. And celery, research shows, has only a little phosphorus.

• That white eggs are healthier than brown—though the fact is that the breed of hen determines egg shell color and the color has nothing to do with nutritive value.

• That vegetable juices are superior to vegetables—when, in fact, nutritive values are the same and whole vegetables form an important source of bulk for the diet.

• That you can expect harmful, even poisonous effects from various food combinations—oysters and ice cream, buttermilk and cabbage, milk and any kind of fish, milk and potatoes, milk and tomatoes, milk and spinach. Yet no evidence from medical experience—or actual test investigations—indicates that such combinations are harmful.

And still other common misconceptions include the

idea that wine makes blood (no single food does); ice water causes heart trouble (no); food left in an opened can is dangerous (not if the can is covered and the food kept cool); and a hot meal is more nourishing than a cold one (purely a matter of taste since temperature doesn't affect nutrient values).

Some false notions still surround the subject of food values for athletes and sportsmen.

Even ten years ago, researchers from the Harvard School of Public Health were pointing out that eating red meat just before a football game may make a player think he is stronger but actually has little physical value. They reported that most of the value of training tables and such foods as rare meat is psychological. The training table—as a type of ritual—helps provide some sense of security and reassurance to the athlete. And giving an athlete special food helps make him feel that his training, which has required hard work and the foregoing of many pleasures, has some "incidental rewards."

The Harvard doctors also noted that the trained athlete really needs no extra protein except during periods of very rigorous training when liberal quantities of protein should be included in the diet in order to allow muscles to increase in size without depriving other parts of the body of the protein they need, too.

Actually, the best diet for an athlete, according to the Harvard researchers, is one that he enjoys and that provides a variety of nutritious foods in amounts adequate to maintain his proper weight.

Yet, only recently—at the 1965 annual meeting of the American College Health Association—Dr. Donald L. Cooper, team physician at Oklahoma State University, declared that "we still see coaches and proponents of athletic endeavor who swear by the heavy-protein or meat-dominated diet."

"It is true," he remarked, "that a certain minimal amount of meat or protein is necessary but this actually should be only a part of a balanced diet and certainly not the dominant part. It is not protein that is burned up; in the final analysis, it is glycogen or simple sugars and phosphates."

In its most recent (1965) handbook on athletic training, the American Medical Association also pointed out:

"Recent research suggests that an emphasis on carbohydrates (sugars and starches) in the diet of the athlete, particularly for endurance events, may be warranted. Also contrary to the traditional ideas, research indicates that 'going heavy' on protein in the training diet serves no useful purpose. These studies show that in strenuous activity there is an increased utilization of carbohydrates if these are available. Protein, as was formerly believed, does not seem to be the chief source of muscular energy."

Says Dr. Cooper: "In terms of efficiency of utilization of oxygen, it must be noted that one liter of oxygen yields five calories if used to burn carbohydrates but only 4.5 calories if used to burn protein or fat. This is a 10 percent difference in the utilization of oxygen and may be an important factor in performance under certain circumstances."

And when it comes to meals before strenuous activities, Dr. Cooper adds, proteins may best be avoided. For when proteins are digested and broken down, an acid is left which can only be removed by the kidneys—but effective kidney function stops during exercise and the acid can't be removed. On the other hand, when the body digests and breaks down carbohydrates—and even fats—carbon dioxide is the main residue. And carbon dioxide can be blown off via the lungs and excreted by the skin.

"Increased acid in the muscles and system in general accounts for fatigue, cramps, and inability to function so it is easy to see why an athlete who eats a large steak, eggs, or other protein meal before a contest can expect more troubles with fatigue and acidosis."

Basics of Nutrition

Five main food components are required by the body —carbohydrates, fats, proteins, vitamins and minerals. While no one food furnishes all, virtually all foods contain several in varying amounts.

While vitamins and minerals are essential to normal body functioning, we get our fuel or energy—and the means for growth and replacement of worn-out tissues— from carbohydrates, fats and proteins.

Carbohydrates are the most plentiful sources of energy and usually furnish up to 50 percent of caloric intake.

Fats are more concentrated sources of calories; ounce for ounce, they yield about twice as many calories as do carbohydrates or proteins.

In the typical American diet, fats provide 40 to 45 percent of calories, and the balance of 10 to 15 percent comes from protein. If weight is above normal, an efficient way to bring it down is to lower fat intake. And for some time nutritionists have been suggesting that

increasingly sedentary Americans would do well to reduce fat intake to about 30 to 35 percent of total calories
as a means of possibly helping to prevent heart trouble.

Particularly in this country, Nature has been bounti-
ful. Achieving good nutrition is easy. Vital nutritional
elements are available in a huge variety of foods. And
if there are some foods you dislike, you don't have to
worry: there are plenty of others to suit your taste
and meet your needs.

A Healthy Food Lineup

A good food lineup to provide all needed carbohydrates, fats, proteins, minerals and vitamins for an adult
would include, daily, foods chosen from these four
groups:

Bread and Cereals: 3 to 4 servings of enriched or
restored bread or cereal (choice of cornmeal, grits, rice,
rolled oats, etc., macaroni, spaghetti, noodles, baked
goods).

Milk: 1 to 2 cups—or the need for nutrients (including calcium for bones and teeth, vitamin A, riboflavin
and many others) in this amount of milk can be satisfied
by cheeses or ice cream (1 cup of milk about equals 1½
cups of cottage cheese or 2–3 scoops of ice cream).

Meat: one large serving of beef, veal, pork, lamb,
poultry, fish or eggs; or, as alternates, dry beans, peas or
nuts.

Vegetables-Fruits: 4 or more daily servings to include
a citrus fruit or other fruit or vegetable high in vitamin
C; other fruits and vegetables including potatoes; and at
least every other day a green or yellow vegetable.

The Cholesterol Business

Nobody knows why but in men the coronary arteries which nourish the heart muscle are favorite sites for atherosclerosis, a building up of fatty deposits. As the deposits accumulate on the inner linings of the coronaries and reduce their bore, coronary insufficiency develops. The heart muscle, its nourishment reduced, becomes less efficient.

As artery clogging increases, *angina pectoris* may develop. This is the agonizing chest pain that appears with exertion and signals that the burden on the heart is too great. Then, at some point, when a blood clot comes along and gets wedged in a narrowed portion of a coronary artery, shutting off blood flow to part of the heart muscle, a heart attack may occur.

Cholesterol is believed to be a factor in atherosclerosis. This soft, waxy yellowish substance is important in the body's chemical functioning. It comes from a wide variety of foods and also is produced in the body by the liver. It circulates through the blood stream.

A statistical correlation between abnormally high levels of cholesterol in the blood and coronary artery disease has been established by many researchers. And investigations have determined that blood cholesterol levels can be lowered by reducing intake of saturated fats such as those found in pork, whole milk, butter and eggs, and foods from other animal sources, and by use of polyunsaturated fats (largely from vegetable oils).

There have also been studies indicating that heart attack incidence is reduced when blood cholesterol levels are brought down to normal. One of the most recent, for example, was conducted by physicians at the Atherosclerosis Research Center, Montclair, N.J. and involved 200 men, aged 20 to 50, who were followed for a five-year period. All 200 already had had heart attacks. One hundred were placed on a diet restricting fat to 30 percent of total calories, with a high proportion in the form of polyunsaturated. The other 100 ate what they liked, presumably a typical American diet containing 40 to 45 percent fat, the bulk of it from animal sources. At the end of the five years, the men in the unrestricted diet group had a heart attack recurrence rate $1\frac{1}{2}$ times greater than the others.

But if cholesterol may be involved, so it seems are other factors. There is clear evidence, as noted earlier, that sedentary living can contribute to development of coronary artery disease and that regular exercise helps reduce its incidence. Evidently, too, exercise (as for the Masai tribesmen, for example) is important in lowering blood cholesterol levels.

The question of exactly how important cholesterol is as a heart disease factor and whether there should be radical changes in the general American diet remains unsettled. Late in 1965 when the American Medical Association's Council on Foods and Nutrition took a hard look at the problem, it noted that there was still no "definitive proof that lowering serum cholesterol, or preventing a rise in serum cholesterol, will lower the morbidity and mortality associated with coronary heart disease." But it did suggest that physicians "consider regulating dietary fat" in young men as a worthwhile possible, even if not definitely proven, means of trying to reduce risks; and it suggested that such regulation may be all the more desirable in men with other factors that increase the likelihood of heart trouble—factors such as high blood pressure, obesity, a positive family history of coronary artery disease. Thus, depending upon circumstances in the individual case, physicians may make specific recommendations about changes in diet.

For the average man, it might well be worthwhile to moderate fat intake if it is presently excessive, to eat perhaps a bit more fish and a bit less meat, some poly-unsaturated margarine on occasion in place of butter, and to use skim milk occasionally in place of whole milk all the time.

If You're Overweight

Desirable weight is basically a matter of balance—correct balance between energy intake and energy expenditure. The plain unvarnished fact is that most overweight people eat more calories than they burn up and the difference is deposited as fat. If food intake equals energy output, weight remains stable. And if excess pounds are present, they'll come off only by making food intake less than energy output.

If you have an excess weight problem, you can go to the extreme of complete fasting. But that's not the best way. The best and safest way is to increase physical activity and couple that with reasonable reduction in food intake.

No less important, you don't have to be a mealtime martyr, a follower of one of the fad diets that keep turning up in infinite variety in newspapers and magazines and books. Usually, they claim to be uniquely successful because of this or that variation in the proportions of calories derived from carbohydrates, fats and proteins. But nutrition experts have found that their success, usually temporary, comes not from a variation but simply from the reduced total calorie intake they require.

"There is no evidence," one scientific report noted recently, "to support the value of any of these variations over that which can result from a diet that is well balanced but reduced in calories. There may result from some of the variations in nutrients a fairly rapid weight loss in the initial period. This has been found, however, to be water loss and not body fat."

Recently, because even physicians sometimes may be confused by the claims made for various methods of dieting, a medical publication asked a top medical nutritionist how he would advise the family doctor to advise any patient who wants to reduce. His reply: He should recommend "that the average patient who wishes to lose weight simply eat less than what he has been eating, assuming he eats a varied diet so as to receive a balanced diet. But he should be specific about the eating less—one piece of toast instead of two, one egg instead of two, a small chocolate sundae instead of a large one, one cocktail instead of two. He should insist that the patient weigh himself weekly at the same time (for example, every Sunday morning before breakfast), and keep a written record of his weight.

"The 'cutting down, not out' and the 'cutting up' (increased physical activity) should be adjusted by the patient so that a weight loss of 1 to 2 pounds per week is attained until desirable weight is reached and then maintained.

"As in many other things in our society, self-discipline and common sense are required for success in weight reduction, not a diet low or high in carbohydrate, fat, protein, or vitamins."

And that's the on-the-line truth—simple, unadorned and valuable. Especially valuable for any outdoorsman who happens to be overweight and wants to get rid of the excess baggage and be fit and healthy too.

10 Eating on the Go

Once the standard for food for the trail was 3 pounds per man per day of beans, bacon and bannock, with the bannock made on the spot from flour. With what game he could get, the three B's kept a man's stomach full.

Today's outdoorsman is more fortunate. With dehydrated foods readily available in any supermarket and more sophisticated sportsman's meals with freeze-dried meats available in many sporting goods stores, eating on the trail can be varied, well-balanced, palatable.

In addition to being light in weight, such foods are compactly packaged, take less space in a pack, allow other conveniences to be carried that otherwise might have to be left behind.

One-Week Grub List

There is no one ideal food list. Just so long as you make up a list that provides a balanced diet—with foods from the four basic groups (milk and milk products, bread and cereals, fruits and vegetables, meat and meat products)—you'll eat well and healthily.

Here, as an example, is a list that makes for a balanced diet, can serve one man for a week, and weighs only 16½ pounds:

Bacon	1 lb.
Powdered eggs	½ lb.
Cereals	1½ lb.
Instant tea or coffee (or, if preferred, chocolate or bouillon cubes)	½ lb.
Sugar	1 lb.
Prepared pancake mix	1 lb.
Salt, pepper, other seasoning	½ lb.
Dried peaches, apples, prunes, other fruit	1½ lb.
Chocolate bars	½ lb.
Dry beans	1 lb.
Powdered milk	1 lb.
Raisins	½ lb.
Dehydrated vegetables	1 lb.
Dried soups in envelopes	½ lb.
Rice	½ lb.
Crackers, pilot biscuits or hardtack	1 lb.
Chipped beef	½ lb.
Cured ham	1½ lb.
Macaroni	½ lb.
Cheese	½ lb.

Chances are you'll be able to add some fresh fish or game for variety.

Two-Week Grub List

As a second example, here is a well-tested basic grub list that can take care of the nutritional needs—and healthy appetite—of one man for two weeks:

Fresh meat (for first day out)	3/4 lb.
Bacon	5 lb.
Butter, canned	1 1/4 lb.
Shortening (Crisco or similar)	1/2 lb.
Dried beef	1/2 lb.
Dry sausage	1 lb.
Cheese	3/4 lb.
Corned beef	1 can
Baked bread (for first day)	1/2 loaf
Wafers (Ry-Krisp or similar)	1 1/2 lb.
Cornmeal or corn-muffin mix	1 1/4 lb.
Rice	1 lb.
Quick-cooking oats	3/4 lb.
Pancake flour	2 1/2 lb.
Plain flour	1 lb.
Biscuit mix	2 lb.
Gingerbread mix	1/2 lb.
Macaroni	1/2 lb.
Baking powder	1/8 lb.
Dried milk	1 1/2 lb.
Dehydrated potatoes	1 lb.
Dehydrated onions	1/8 lb.
Dehydrated carrots	1/8 lb.
Dried eggs	1/4 lb.
Dehydrated soup	1/2 lb.
Split dried peas	1/8 lb.

Coffee	1 lb.
Tea	⅛ lb.
Cocoa	¼ lb.
Sugar	4 lb.
Pudding mix	2 packages
Jam or jelly	1 lb.
Candy bars	2 lb.
Salt	½ lb.
Dry beans	1½ lb.
Dried fruit	2½ lb.
Tomatoes	2 cans
Pepper	1 oz.
Cinnamon	1 oz.
Baking soda	1 oz.
Powdered lemon juice	½ lb.

Your Own List

Selecting items from all four basic food groups, you can make up a grub list to suit your taste and the tastes of others in your party.

In making up a list, it's a good idea—and many outdoorsmen get an anticipatory kick out of doing so in preparation for a trip—to write out menus. That way, you can plan for variety and how much of each item to pack.

If you haven't the time or inclination to figure out all menus in advance, planning those for one day will give you some idea of quantities needed for one day and, by multiplication, total quantities for the trip.

The point is to plan—by whatever system you wish to use—for well-balanced (and preferably varied and interesting) eating on the trail rather than head for a super-market and make random choices until you have a load you hope will do the trick and, more likely than not, will prove inadequate.

Sweets and Vitamins

You will have noticed that both of the sample grub lists include candy bars. It's a good idea to have choco-late or, if you prefer, hard candy along to provide quick energy.

Do you need vitamins? A balanced diet usually sup-plies all the vitamins you need. But on an extended trip with dehydrated rations, even though you're not likely to suffer from any undue deficiencies, it could be help-ful to take along vitamins.

Dish Sanitation

Nuisance it may be, but keeping every item you cook in and eat out of scrupulously clean can make the differ-ence between a rewarding trip and one full of gripes.

Microorganisms capable of producing mild abdomi-nal upsets at best and some pretty severe ones at worst can multiply quickly when they can feed on little scraps of food left on plates and utensils.

And you don't even have to have microorganisms to cause trouble. For example, grease left in an improperly scoured skillet may absorb lye from soapy dishwater and cause a gastrointestinal unpleasantness next time food is prepared.

It's easier to get grease out of a skillet while it's still warm. Household detergents aren't as easy to carry as a solid cake of soap—but they have their merits. They work well in all kinds of water, cut grease fast, are easy to rinse off. Worthwhile taking: a little scouring pad.

The hotter the water, the easier it is to wash dishes. And dishes rinsed in hot water don't have to be wiped dry. Put a kettle of water over the fire as soon as you've finished preparing a meal and it will be boiling hot and ready for use by the time you're finished eating.

Divide the water between two pails. Add soap or detergent to one and use it for washing. Rinse in the clear water. It's a good idea to keep the latter boiling over the fire and to dip the soapy dishes in it.

Pure Water

The higher you go in wilderness country, the more likely water will be pure, uncontaminated by man. That's especially true when you get to mountain springs and creek beginnings. But you can never be absolutely certain these days. You can be suspicious, of course, when water has a peculiar odor. But there is no 100 percent sure way of detecting contamination other than by chemical analysis. And although many people have used polluted water for drinking without harm, it's a gamble hardly worth taking.

There are several ways to purify questionable water.

Boiling it for at least five minutes is one. There will be a flat taste but you can offset that if you pour the water back and forth a few times between two containers to restore the air lost during boiling. Some people like to sprinkle in a bit of salt as an extra measure for overcoming the flat taste.

Instead of boiling you can use chemicals. Chlorine tablets for water purification are available at drug stores and come with instructions for use. Tincture of iodine—about 2 or 3 drops per quart—will make water safe. Also available in drug and sporting goods stores are halazone tablets which do a quick job of germ killing. They cost little more than aspirin tablets, come in bottles with instructions for use. After chemical treatment, water should be allowed to stand for at least half an hour before you drink it.

Natural Foods

Unless you really know your mushrooms, don't pick them. They haven't enough food value to warrant taking the risk of picking a deadly variety.

But there are many kinds of natural foods which, if you're broad-minded enough, can be used if you should ever have a food emergency—and also on occasion to add some variety to the grub you pack.

For example, any snake, including a poisonous one (the poison is in sacs in the head not in edible meat in the body), can be nourishing. Some people prize snake meat, and lizard meat as well. The chicken is an edible bird—but so is the crow and just about any other bird. And the eggs of any bird can help contribute to a meal.

Not only are grasshoppers nourishing; the Japanese consider them a delicacy. And if you eat a porcupine or a muskrat in an emergency, you'll satisfy your hunger and possibly run a risk of developing a liking.

The list of wild plants a man can eat and be nourished by is almost endless. There are, of course, the wild berries—blueberries, raspberries, cranberries, huckle-berries. Wild rice, if you can find it, is a treasure. Water-lily bulbs, dandelions, pigweed, plantain, fern sprouts—all are edible.

Boil grass and it makes a nourishing green. You can boil and eat cattail and camas roots.

There are a few poisonous plants and fruits. And one experienced outdoorsman suggests two rules to follow that will almost certainly keep you out of trouble with them:

1. Steer clear of any unidentified fruit, plant stem or tuber that contains a white, milklike fluid.

2. If a strange plant food after being cooked stings or burns your mouth when you take a small sample taste, don't eat it.

Part II

PREPARING FOR SPECIAL
AREAS AND SITUATIONS

11 High Altitudes

So thin is the air in the last quarter of the climb to Mt. Everest's 29,028-foot summit that human muscle, nerves and mental processes deteriorate. Even tying a shoelace becomes a herculean job as muscles seem to become glued by fatigue and the head splits.

So reports Dr. Gilbert Roberts, 28-year-old former Air Force surgeon who was one of the members and senior medical officer of the American expedition that scaled the Himalayan peak in the spring of 1963.

"No one," Roberts says, "can realize the terrible conditions faced by man at that altitude. It's just dragging one incredibly weary foot after another . . . every man noticeably deteriorating day after day, fighting for air, pushing one more step upward against muscles that can't, but must, perform. It's minds that beg to quit, with warmth and decent sleep a distant memory."

Yet Everest gets scaled. And there is evidence from an experiment by famed climber Sir Edmund Hillary that, given time, man can acclimate himself to very high altitudes so they no longer are agonizingly tough to take.

In the autumn of 1961, Hillary and a group of climbers built a hut in the Himalayas at an altitude of 19,000 feet. Supplied with warm clothes, an oil stove, all the food they needed, they spent the winter there, seeking to adapt themselves to the height with its oxygen rarity.

They succeeded. The oxygen content of their blood dropped day after day. Yet they soon could carry out almost as hard physical work as at lower altitudes. Ordinarily, a healthy man not used to rarefied air would become a victim of hypoxia, or oxygen deficiency, unable to function at all, when the oxygen content of his blood drops significantly.

The chances are not many readers of this book will be trying to climb Mt. Everest or to work for extended periods at heights of 19,000 feet or above. But much lower altitudes can affect performance.

For several years now, because the 1968 Olympics are to be held in Mexico City with its altitude of 2,250 meters (about 7,000 feet), physiologists, sports physicians and other scientists have been conducting extensive investigations of how moderate altitudes affect physical efficiency and how best to prepare for performing at such altitudes. Some of the information they have been getting will be useful to outdoorsmen who have occasion to hunt or engage in other activities at moderately high altitudes.

Effects of Moderate Altitude

In the summer of 1964, Dr. Bruno Balke of the University of Wisconsin carried out controlled experiments with a group of well-trained athletes, first at Oklahoma City (400 meters elevation) and then at Red River, New Mexico (2,300 meters).

Shortly after their arival at Red River, all the subjects showed a reduced oxygen intake capacity in comparison to measurements made in Oklahoma City. In almost all cases, however, as they worked out and became accustomed to the mountains over a two-week period, oxygen intake capacity returned to nearly normal:

When it came to sprint-type efforts—400-meter events —performance remained practically unaffected by altitude. That had been expected because it's known that breathing difficulty occurs after, not during, short, sprint-type activities. It was also expected—and found— that since a given volume of air at higher altitudes contains fewer molecules of oxygen, recovery after a sprint would take longer than at sea level.

On the other hand, mile runs at Red River were notably slower than at Oklahoma City. In a mile run or other endurance activity, muscle tissue requires a continuous and adequate supply of oxygen. Even at 2,000 meters elevation, the reduced amount of oxygen in the air can slightly lower the amount of oxygen in the arterial blood. If the heart and lungs could work harder, they could compensate but usually they are already functioning at their maximum during an endurance event.

When a similar experiment was repeated in 1965, results were much the same. For example, Jack Daniels, a former Olympian and the best conditioned of the subjects, ran a 2:19 half-mile his first week at altitude as against a sea-level time of 2:13. His time for the mile increased from 5:00 to 5:23 and for 2½ miles from 13:42 to 14:45. During his second week at altitude, he did the half-mile in 2:14 and the mile in 5:13. But there was no gain during the third week, with Daniels running the half-mile in 2:15 and the mile again in 5:13.

Overall, the two summers of experiments revealed a 5 to 6 percent difference in performance at sea level and altitude.

Fitness and Altitude Tolerance

Of even more direct interest to many outdoorsmen are the results of studies showing how valuable getting into good physical shape can be in increasing tolerance for high-altitude conditions. Conducted for three consecutive summers by Dr. Cutting B. Favour of Denver and reported in the spring of 1966, the studies were supported by the Army's Medical Research and Development Command.

The subjects were healthy but sedentary men. Many were young men, 25 years or younger, a number of them medical students. There were older men—the oldest, 52.

All were subjected to a battery of tests on four occasions—first at low altitude, then during a week's exposure to the 14,150-foot altitude of Mount Evans, again at low altitude after a month-long physical conditioning program, and then again during a week's stay on Mount Evans.

During the month-long conditioning period, the subjects worked out at least an hour daily for five days a week, and most of them also engaged in weekend physical activities.

While a "longer fitness program would be desirable," Dr. Favour reported, it was significant that "a sedentary, healthy man can benefit greatly from an exercise program as short and as simple as the one used in the study."

The measure of lactic acid in the blood after activity

indicates the degree of fitness. The fitter the man, the lower the lactic acid level. The study showed that the lactic acid level was lower, both at low and high altitude, in the men after they became fit. While there was some deterioration in overall physical performance at altitude, it was far less in the fit state.

Furthermore, measurements showed a lesser need for oxygen during strenuous activity at altitude during the fit state than during the sedentary. Ability to use oxygen efficiently evidently increased. It was also notable that fit subjects had fewer episodes of any kind of discomforting symptoms at altitude.

In presenting his conclusions at an International Symposium on the Effects of Altitude on Physical Performance, Dr. Favour declared that the fit subject "can perform useful effort when the sedentary subject may not be able to work at all."

Mountain Sickness

The outdoorsman going off to high-altitude country on a hunting, skiing or other trip can expect that if he conditions himself with the program offered earlier in this book, he will experience relatively little deterioration in strength and endurance and is less likely to have to wage a constant battle against fatigue. He is also less likely to develop mountain sickness.

A miserable affliction, mountain sickness produces such symptoms as headache, nausea, vomiting, dizziness, diarrhea and generalized weakness. In some cases, there may be only two or three symptoms; in the more severe cases, all may appear.

What causes it? Often, it stems simply from excessive effort—too great demand placed on the body which isn't accustomed to strenuous activity. It's far less likely to originate this way if you're in good physical condition.

But there are other possible causes that have to be considered. It is believed that hiking or climbing too rapidly may be a factor. So, too, becoming either overheated or too cold.

If mountain sickness does occur, the symptoms usually disappear within a few days. If you're unlucky enough to experience them and they persist, better get home and see your physician since something more serious could be involved.

A More Dangerous Form

There is a much more serious, even potentially fatal, disorder which may affect sedentary men who suddenly rush off to high altitudes and engage in strenuous activity. It was identified in 1964 in two skiers, both of them physicians. Chances are it has produced fatalities in the past which have been attributed to other causes. It's called "acute pulmonary edema of altitude" and involves water-logging of the lungs.

The two physicians who experienced near-fatal attacks were normally healthy men living sedentary lives who, most of the year, got little more exercise than what is involved in making hospital rounds and playing weekend golf. Both were skiing enthusiasts and had rushed from their low-elevation offices to the nearly 11,000-foot high slopes of Utah's Alta ski resort and had immediately, without wasting a moment, set out skiing in heavy, fresh wet spring snow.

After two days, they became intensely ill, had great difficulty in breathing. Their symptoms suggested some sort of heart disease or pneumonia or both. Close to death, they were brought down to an altitude of 4,500 feet, hospitalized in Salt Lake City where they recovered with bed rest and oxygen treatment.

X-ray studies showed that the lungs of both men were filled with fluids squeezed out of the blood vessels into the air spaces of the lungs. Other studies indicated that this was caused by spasm—involuntary contractions—of blood vessels leading from lungs to heart.

One of the medical investigators who studied and reported these cases is Dr. Hans H. Hecht, Professor of Medicine at the University of Utah College of Medicine and an accomplished skier himself. He believes that "the kind of overexertion experienced in high-altitude skiing by a relatively sedentary person is likely to bring out this condition in nearly any susceptible person."

Dr. Hecht advises sedentary men going in for high-altitude skiing to take several precautions:

Spend at least a day or two after arriving at the ski lodge taking it easy and getting acclimatized to the high altitude.

When skiing in earnest starts, break up the day with a leisurely lunch. Eight to twelve hours of vigorous skiing by an unprepared man could lead to trouble unless interrupted some way.

If shortness of breath or labored breathing becomes noticeable, stop skiing for the day and go to a lower elevation. If this is not possible, see a physician and get some pure oxygen.

Outdoorsmen on hunting or other trips to high altitude areas would do well to take similar precautions. Especially if you're not in top physical condition, give yourself some time to get acclimated before you go all-out—and break up a vigorous day with rest periods. It's good advice to follow even if you are in peak condition and therefore likely to be less susceptible to trouble.

The Sunburn Problem

A severe case of sunburn is never a joke—and sunburn can be particularly severe at high altitude. That's because the sun's ultraviolet rays are far more intense there. You can get severely sunburned even when air temperature is well below freezing.

Unless you start out with a good protective coat of tan, it's a good idea to carry along and use a preparation to help screen out some of the ultraviolet. There are many such preparations on the market.

Avoid using excessive amounts of soap on your face; stick to the minimum needed for washing. Soap tends to remove natural oils that help protect the skin from sun.

Some experienced outdoorsmen who know their high-altitude conditions make a habit of carrying a chapstick in a pocket and applying it to the lips and nostrils as a means of countering sunlight reflected upward from snow which often affects these areas most.

Snowblindness

It doesn't take long before glaring light makes the eyes start burning and watering. It may even make them see double.

There can be plenty of glare at high altitudes from the sun—and also from light reflected by snow. Snow, in fact, can reflect enough light even with overcast skies to cause trouble.

Carry along—and use—dark glasses. Get the best you can afford—and consider the type with side shields which provide extra protection.

12   Cold Regions

Recently more and more sportsmen have been making hunting and camping trips to Alaska and Northern Canada and to areas of the United States where the weather can be very cold, sometimes not much less so than in polar regions.

Extreme cold isn't tough to take if you're prepared to cope with it properly. And recent research—some of it supported by the Army—has been producing information that can be useful to any outdoorsman planning an excursion into cold-weather country.

The research has been demonstrating that although man is essentially a semitropical animal, some peoples have been able to make very special, surprising adapations to extreme cold; that while most of us today can't make such special adaptations, we do after a time adapt otherwise; that we don't have to depend upon any special kinds of foods to get along well in extreme cold; that the critical factor in staying healthy and comfortable is clothing—both the right kind and its proper use.

The Business of Adaptation

Ever since the young Charles Darwin 130 years ago visited Tierra del Fuego at the southern tip of South America and found the Yahgan Indians living there virtually naked, physiologists have been puzzled by the stamina of certain racial groups in polar environments.

Darwin reported that as his ship, the *Beagle*, landed in a flurry of mid-winter sleet, Indians came out in canoes, apparently indifferent to the wet and cold. Primarily fishermen, the Yahgans kept their boats moored offshore in kelp beds and took chilly swims to shore without appearing to mind.

Recently new understanding about human adaptability to cold has come from the work of Dr. Per F. Scholander, professor of physiology at the University of California's Scripps Institution of Oceanography at La Jolla.

In a special study of Australian aborigines, Dr. Scholander found a situation similar to that which existed among the Yahgans. For a long time, the aborigines lived without clothing in the coldest parts of the continent. The custom lasted generally until just a few decades ago but even now, Dr. Scholander found, natives are likely to discard their clothes entirely on hunting expeditions or use them as pillows at night. Although temperatures on winter nights fall below freezing, they keep warm by sleeping on the ground between small campfires.

To study the aborigines' ability to live this way with cold, Scholander and a group of scientists went to Australia, taking along instruments, thermocouples, that could be placed on the skin at various sites to make scientific measurements.

The scientists first compared their own ability to sleep nude between the small campfires with that of the natives. They found that on windless nights, they could endure the conditions if they constantly attended the fires; they got little sleep. On windy nights, the situation was unbearable. Yet the natives slept well with only occasional attention to the fires.

When measurements were made with the thermo-couples, they showed that skin temperatures of the natives were much lower than those of the scientists. At times, skin areas shielded from the fire heat got down to 54 degrees F, yet the natives didn't wake up.

In another test, scientists and natives spent a night nude in lightweight sleeping bags, each the equivalent of a single blanket. There were no fires. The natives slept comfortably while the scientists shivered and stayed awake most of the night. Skin temperatures on the scientists' feet fell to 59 degrees; they fell even further on the natives' feet but they went on sleeping.

Shivering produces heat. But the natives didn't shiver. Nor was there any increase in their metabolic or heat-production rate during the night. Apparently they had developed a striking ability to tolerate low temperatures without enough discomfort to keep them awake and without need for increasing their body heat production.

Civilized man can adapt to cold but does it a different way, perhaps because he has so long used clothes and shelter, Dr. Scholander has been able to show.

One striking example of the latter type of adaptation came during the ill-fated Hubbard expedition into Labrador in 1903. While Hubbard himself died, his two companions walked for two months in deep snow until they finally reached safety. On the way, they lost their shoes, most of their warm clothes, had the use of only half a blanket each at night. When they got back to civilization, they felt stifled in warm houses, had to go outside every so often "to breathe."

To investigate this type of adaptation, Dr. Scholander went into the mountains of Norway for six weeks with eight Norwegian college students as volunteer subjects. They wore lightweight summer clothing—down to cotton shorts, adding only a light parka and cotton trousers when it got very cold. At night they slept naked in one-blanket sleeping bags like those in the Australian aboriginese experiment.

For the first few nights, they had trouble sleeping, kept thrashing around trying to get warm. After a week, however, they were sleeping comfortably. At the end of the experiment, thermocouple measurements showed that at night, in the sleeping bags, the feet of the students, unlike the aborigines, stayed warm. The students had adapted by increasing body heat production, rather than by learning to tolerate cold.

According to Dr. Scholander, anyone who goes on a camping trip in the high mountains or other cold territory can expect that he will begin to adapt. He won't be able to do it as primitive peoples do it by learning how to remain reasonably comfortable while body temperature falls. But he'll get some comfort as his metabolism goes up and his body produces more heat.

For practical purposes, however, the comfort that comes from adaptation is limited and secondary. The prime factor is clothing.

Clothing

Not long ago, when the World Health Organization held a special conference on health and cold climate conditions, it was attended by physicians, anthropologists, nutritionists, physiologists and other scientists. Out of it came general agreement that man can live normally—very well, indeed—even in polar regions.

To do so he doesn't need any special diet. Eskimos, the conferees noted, do not eat seal and walrus blubber to keep warm. They eat it because it is available, because it is an excellent, nutritionally balanced food—and because they like it.

A man living in the cold needs neither extra fats, proteins nor carbohydrates to stay warm. What he does need, the scientists emphasized, is good clothing which can protect the physiologic climate contained by his skin.

Even at rest, the body is continuously producing heat. When you lose heat to the surrounding air at the same rate as it is produced, you feel comfortable. Lose more heat than is being generated and you feel cold.

The purpose of clothing, of course, is to reduce the rate of heat loss in cold weather. It achieves this by insulating body surfaces from cold air, keeping them dry, and sheltering them from wind.

For extreme cold, the fur clothing of the Eskimo is excellent—capable, the WHO conference established, of providing virtually as much warmth as a well-heated house. Immediately next to his skin, the Eskimo wears newborn caribou fur, hair side in. On top of this, he wears a heavier layer, hair side out.

When it set out to develop better clothes for Arctic troops, the U.S. Army Quartermaster Corps thoroughly investigated the Eskimo costume. It discovered that caribou had no special qualities as an insulating material.

The studies established that caribou and other furs—and virtually all insulating materials—generally provide about 4 clos of insulation per inch of thickness. A clo is defined as the insulation needed to keep a man comfortable in a 70-degree environment.

The studies indicated that virtually all the insulating value in any material comes not from the material itself but from dead air. An inch of air is actually worth seven clos. It has to be trapped, though—and the fabric or hairs used to trap it somewhat reduce the air's insulating effectiveness. And the research established that trapped air is most effective in clothing of quarter-inch thickness.

Out of this work came the Army's cold-weather clothing system which involves the use of many layers of light and loose garments instead of just one or two heavy ones. In a nutshell, the more such garments, the more free insulation you get—via the slices of air trapped between the garments.

Wind Chill

Other important research has been concerned with the effect of wind chill. If you're standing outdoors with the temperature, say, at about 23, the air still, and you're only lightly clad, you may feel cool but not miserably cold. If the sun should happen to be shining brightly, you may even feel pleasant at this temperature.

But if a wind should spring up, you would feel definitely cold when the velocity reached 1 to 2 miles per hour. At about 4 mph, you'd be very cold. At about 9 mph, you would be bitterly cold even though the temperature hadn't changed one degree.

It takes only a 2 to 3 mile per hour wind to make the skin cool at a rate twice that when air is moving at less than 1 mile per hour. With a rise in wind velocity from zero to 4 mph, you get about the same cooling effect as from a 10-degree temperature drop.

Wind exerts a chilling effect by disturbing stagnant air layers over the skin and between garments. And because it works this way, wind chill may have its maximum effect when wind velocity is relatively low and you may be wearing little clothing.

Thus it's always important to carry with you—even for moderate climates—an outer garment of windproof fabric. A thin windbreaker often can do as much to keep you warm as a much thicker insulation layer.

As for other garments to take along on trips into cold areas, you can select them to suit your own taste, keeping in mind just a few basic guidelines:

1. The first layer immediately next to the skin should be loose-fitting to trap air, and also to allow some ventilation when you move about and thus begin to increase body heat production.

2. Over the first layer, you can wear as many additional layers—including another of underwear, one or more shirts, etc.—as you need to keep warm. They don't have to be heavy and bulky; they can be light and they should be loose.

3. You should be able to put on and take off the layers readily as needed.

Proper Use

That last point—easy on and off—is important and can even be critical in cold-weather country. Sitting still, a man produces only about as much heat as a 75-watt light bulb—an amount known technically as a metabolic unit. When he does very light work—at a machine, for example—he may produce double that amount of heat. Walking briskly he can generate four units—and if he is carrying a 45-pound pack at a brisk pace he may produce 6 units.

Thus the layers needed to insulate and keep him warm when he is sitting still will be too many when he is active. And the great danger lies in getting overheated and working up a sweat.

In a cold climate, sweating is dangerous because the moisture accumulates in the clothing. Wet clothing isn't just uncomfortable because it's wet; it loses its insulation value. The water—or ice—fills up the trapped air spaces.

When you're active in a cold climate, take care to prevent overheating. As you move from inactivity to activity, anticipate the effects of the latter. You may start by pushing back your hood and opening your clothes at neck and wrists. If, after this, your activity is strenuous enough to make you still feel on the warm side, remove an outer garment. Remove still more if necessary to keep you from sweating. When your activity slows, add a garment. When you stop working entirely, get all dressed up again. If you try to keep reasonably cool, the chances are you'll be warmer in the long run. And while you may spend a lot of time changing clothing layers, it's worth it.

The Head

Even at room temperature, researchers report, as much as 25 percent of total heat lost by the body may be dissipated through the head. According to some calculations, at 40 below, the head alone can get rid of just about all the heat produced by the body of an inactive man.

In a very cold environment, the body, as part of its protective mechanism for trying to conserve heat, may reduce blood flow to the hands and the feet and much of the total skin area but, because of the needs of the brain, it keeps blood flowing at all times to the head.

Obvious moral: Keep your head well protected.

Down to about zero, a wool bill cap with earflaps may be adequate. For below zero weather, many outdoorsmen find a trooper style hat made of fur and fabric, with fold-up earflaps and forehead piece, effective. Also useful for subzero cold: a combination of hooded parka and wool stocking or bill cap.

Hands and Feet

These are special problem areas. The trouble with the hands is that the fingers, shaped much like small cylinders, have an extensive surface area through which heat can be dissipated. And it is difficult to wrap enough insulation around the fingers without making them almost useless.

Mittens are better than gloves since they combine the fingers into a larger volume that can be insulated more effectively. But the trouble with many mittens, investigators have established, is that they are cut so they lie flat. Then, whenever you have to flex a hand, the motion tightens the mitten across the back of the hand, stretching and thinning the insulation. Ideally, you should use a mitten cut to fit a curved hand.

But even the best mittens may not keep your hands warm for more than a few hours at 10 below zero if you're not active. To keep your hands warm, exercise them at frequent intervals or put them inside your clothing whenever you can.

The feet are particularly vulnerable. For one thing, they may get wet often from walking in water or snow and even from perspiration. Also, circulation to the lower extremities is not always as efficient as to other parts of the body so they get less internal heat.

Many experts advise use of two or more pairs of heavy socks and a loose-fitting boot and insole. For cold, wet areas, a waterproof boot is useful. If you're going to be in a dry, cold climate, a felt boot may prove to be warmer than the waterproofed type because it permits moisture to escape.

Trench foot, also called immersion foot, is something to guard against. It results from prolonged cold, short of freezing. In early stages, the feet and toes begin to feel cold, stiff and numb; they have a pale, almost bloodless look. Later, they will swell, become very painful. In extreme cases, the flesh dies and amputation is necessary.

With a few precautions, you can avoid trench foot. And if you act promptly in early stages if it should begin to develop—before pain sets in—you can prevent serious consequences. Keep your feet as dry as possible. Every chance you get, clean and dry shoes and socks.

Any time you get your feet wet, lose no time not only in drying them but also warming them with your hands. If you're in a situation where you can't stop immediately when you wet your feet, exercise them by wriggling your toes, bending your ankles.

Frostbite

Frostbite is the destruction of tissue by freezing. There is always some risk of it in very cold climates, especially when the wind is strong. While there may be considerable pain if hands or feet become frostbitten, that isn't necessarily the case when nose, cheeks or ears are affected.

You can, however, see some of the early effects of frostbite—grayish-white spots on the skin—before you can feel them and the spots serve as a good warning. Keep on the watch for them, and it's a good idea to have a companion keep watch for you while you do the same for him.

A wool face mask can be a protective help in a biting wind. Another good defense for the face is the body heat that collects in the front of a parka hood. It's a considerable help, too, to move your facial muscles at frequent intervals and move your ears with your hands. And don't forget to keep wriggling your fingers and toes.

Frozen spots can be detected not only by sight but also through moving face muscles, ears, fingers and toes and feeling any hardening areas or recognizing any that are becoming numb. Thaw the spots immediately, using your hands and, if necessary, having a companion help with his.

13   The Desert

Trips into desert country appear to be attracting more and more outdoorsmen. Some go desert camping for a look at the flora and fauna; a few, the rock hounds, go to scrabble about for semiprecious stones; some enjoy photographic hunting. In season, hunters may enjoy good bird, deer and other shooting, and anglers find the fishing excellent in Arizona and Nevada along the Colorado River.

North American deserts can be as tough as those anywhere in the world. Is the Sahara hot? The great American Mojave is scarcely less so, with an official maximum temperature of 134 degrees, just .4 less than for the Sahara.

The Variations

If you're going into the desert and want to come back in good health, it's smart to be prepared for weather of almost every conceivable kind. Not just dry heat. Cloudbursts, thunderstorms and hailstones are certainly not everyday occurrences in desert country but they are hardly unknown. After twenty years in which no rain had fallen in July and August in Monument Valley, Arizona, it showered every afternoon through one whole recent summer.

During winter months, most of the world's great

deserts are cool and not infrequently cold. Winter temperatures in the Gobi of Mongolia, for example, go below zero. The Sahara, hot enough from May to October, can be winter-ish from December through February, and ice has been known to form in water pails in March.

Diurnal variations are considerable, too. In a low-latitude desert such as the Sahara, when the temperature shoots above 120 at midday, it can drop to the relatively cool 80's very quickly after sunset and, before morning, may fall to 70 or less.

The Heat Problem

Anyone who has ever felt the direct rays of the sun beating down on him, coming strong through the dry desert air, and has felt the heat bouncing back at him from sand and from rock, isn't likely to forget the experience. If you're in the desert in summer, shelter during the day is a prime requirement.

All desert animals know enough to avoid the midday sun and heat, remaining in the shade of hills or rocks, or burrowing a foot or more underground and sleeping out the day. Experts advise resting in the shade during the hottest part of the day, doing most of your work or traveling by night.

Records of military men under desert conditions indicate that, if you're hiking, you can cover twice the distance on a given amount of water if you move by night rather than by day. It has been figured that the average man hiking in desert country in summer needs one gallon of water for each twenty miles he covers at night; in the sun, a gallon will last him only ten miles.

Natives of the world's great deserts have learned to make use of tents that can be opened at the bottom on all sides to permit free circulation of air during the day and then can be closed at night to conserve heat.

Experts have this advice to offer if you're caught unprepared in the desert:

If your car breaks down, stay in its shade. You may find natural shade on the lee side of a hill, or the overhanging bank of a dry stream bed.

You can improvise a lean-to for shelter with any fabric you have available and any desert growth you can find. For want of other shelter, dig a sand trench deep enough to shade you as you lie in it during the heat of the day. Shade can make as much as a 36-degree difference.

And if no shade is available, the air about a foot above the ground—at the elevation provided by a cot or thick bed of brush—will be many degrees cooler than what you'll find it to be if you sit or lie directly on the ground.

Water

Nothing is more important to the outdoorsman going into the desert or into any hot area than a clear understanding of the facts about the body's need for water.

The human body has been described as a quantity of water surrounded by skin—an apt description since about 60 percent of body weight is water. Water pervades every organ, assists in all vital processes. Blood, urine, sweat, tears and digestive juices are water fluids.

Water is more essential to the body than is food. Lying quietly in a cool area, you might survive ten days without drinking. On the other hand, if given enough water, you could live more than a month without food.

Studies show that the body can lose practically its entire store of starch and fat, even half its protein, without seriously endangering life. But a 10 percent loss of water would prove serious and a 20 percent loss would be dangerous.

Actually, one of the most essential jobs of water—under ordinary circumstances and especially in hot environments—is to keep us cool enough to live, to prevent us from being burned up by the heat the body produces.

Normal body temperature is 98.6 degrees. People have survived falls in body temperature, after exposure, to 78 and even 68 degrees. But death may follow rapidly after a rise of only 10 degrees above normal.

The body cooling system is finely adjusted to keep temperature at normal—and has to be. For even when we're relaxed, feet up and doing nothing, we produce heat. "As long as we live," as one biologist likes to put it, "we are burning as steadily as any flame, sometimes fast, sometimes slowly, according to the circumstances of the moment."

The chief means by which excess heat is removed are exhalation of moisture from the lungs and evaporation of sweat from the skin. When environmental temperature reaches 120, you can lose as much as 2½ pints of sweat in an hour just sitting still.

What's lost must be replaced. If it isn't, you first lose efficiency. Research with men working in desert areas has shown that with loss of about 2 quarts of water—

about 2½ percent of body weight—efficiency drops by 25 percent.

What Happens when You Dehydrate

Research has established a definite progression of symptoms as water is lost and not replaced.

When you first begin to dehydrate—to the extent of 1 to 2 percent of body weight—you feel thirsty and experience vague general discomfort. Soon your movements begin to slow. Appetite diminishes. As you lose more water, you get sleepy, your skin flushes, your pulse rate increases, and you become impatient and irritable. By the time you've lost 5 percent of body weight of water, you're feeling actively nauseous.

As loss continues, getting up to 6 to 10 percent of body weight, you experience dizziness, headache, labored breathing. Soon you feel a tingling in the limbs. Before long, the flow of saliva stops, the body begins to turn blue, speech becomes indistinct.

When the loss reaches 11 percent and beyond, you go into delirium. Your tongue becomes swollen, you are unable to swallow, you lose your hearing, your vision dims, your skin shrivels and then becomes numb, and you may stop urinating.

When does a man die of dehydration? It depends upon the individual—and very much upon air temperature. At an air temperature below 85 degrees, it may be possible for a man to lose as much as 25 percent of body weight in water and still survive. At temperatures above 90, death may occur when dehydration reaches 15 percent.

Drinking and Thirst

Under ordinary circumstances, it takes at the very least 1½ pints of water a day to keep alive. In hot weather, a bare minimum may be a gallon.

Exactly how much you need to prevent dehydration in the desert will depend upon temperature, shelter, activities. Clothing, especially light-colored, helps by reflecting some of the heat of the sun, reducing the amount of sweating. If you stay in the shade as much as possible, take it deliberately very easy when you work, you'll need less water.

With plenty of water—as much as 3 gallons a day—you may be able to work as hard as you like. Provided you can drink the water as often as you like—and drink it even more often than you may like.

If you're active in extremely hot weather, it's a good rule not to depend upon thirst alone to tell you when to drink; if you do, you may begin to dehydrate slowly. Ordinarily, a normal person can rely safely on his sense of thirst to tell him to drink enough water to meet his body requirements. But when a lot of water is suddenly lost through excessive perspiring, the dictates of thirst often may replace only one-half to two-thirds the amount of water lost.

Drink more—and more often—than your thirst tells you to and you'll greatly improve your chances for remaining efficient and warding off fatigue.

Salt

When you sweat profusely, you need to replace not only the water lost but the salt as well. In each quart of sweat, two to four grams of salt are lost. A normal daily diet provides 10 to 12 grams and adequately replaces the salt lost by normal perspiration. But profuse sweating requires additional salt intake.

If salt is not replaced, heat prostration or heat cramps may develop. Heat prostration may begin with warning symptoms of weakness, dizziness, headache, dim or blurred vision, mild muscular cramps. Then the skin becomes ashen, cold and wet, perspiration is profuse, blood pressure falls and in severe cases the victim may become unconscious.

Heat cramps can be excruciating. The victim may become prostrate with legs drawn up or may thrash about, grimacing and sometimes crying out from the pain.

It is possible to replace excessive amounts of salt lost simply by using a little more salt on your food regularly while in hot country than you usually do. It's a good idea to take with you salt tablets and make use of them from time to time, too.

If Water Runs Low

Despite the best planning, emergencies occur. There simply is no substitue for water. Chewing gum or holding a small, smooth pebble at the side of the tongue may offer some relief for a dry mouth—but it adds no water to the system.

If you run short and have to start rationing water, waste no time in rationing your sweat as well. It becomes all the more essential then to shelter yourself as much as possible from the sun, to keep activities to the bare minimum, to perform them in the coolest part of the day and in slow motion.

Keep a lookout for wild berries. Most are edible and high in water content.

Some cacti contain small amounts of water. If you chop into a barrel cactus and eat the pulp, you'll get some moisture. The prickly pear cactus has moisture in the pulp under its spines; you can chew the pulp, suck out the moisture, spit the dry pulp out.

The New Survival Technique

The fact is that even ground which apears to be completely dry may contain some water. At the surface, the water vaporizes into the atmosphere—and, as the vaporized water leaves the soil, some more is drawn up by capillary action. In effect, what the new technique does is to catch the vapor and turn it back into collectable water.

Developed by two U.S. Department of Agriculture research scientists, Drs. Ray D. Jackson and Cornelius H. M. van Bavel, it requires very simple materials: a 6-foot square sheet of clear plastic and a dime-store plastic bucket (or in a pinch an empty coffee can).

It calls for digging a hole about 3 feet across in a sunny spot, placing the bucket at the bottom, covering the hole with the plastic sheet, weighting the edges of the sheet with some dirt, then placing a small rock in the middle of the sheet to weight it down there so it forms an inverted cone.

This is what happens:

As the sun beats down, it raises the temperature of air

and soil under the plastic and speeds up vaporization of water from the soil. The air under the plastic reaches a saturation point; it can't hold any more water vapor. The vapor then begins to condense, forming tiny drops on the undersurface of the plastic. The drops trickle down the sloping underside of the plastic and drip off into the bucket.

And the process doesn't come to a halt at sunset. With the sun gone, there is cooling—but the plastic cools rapidly while the soil temperature stays relatively high. Condensation of water vapor on the undersurface of the plastic continues—not at the same pace as during the day, but the two USDA scientists find they can get about half as much water from 4 P.M. to 8 A.M. as during daylight hours.

Just how much water can such a device—a kind of survival still—produce? In the Arizona desert, not far from Phoenix, plastic-covered water holes have produced up to 2 quarts a day each. Some spots yield less than others. A site that happens to be above underlying rock may soon run out of moisture. But even the poorest location will produce some water. Lowest yield has been a little under a pint a day.

Making the Still

Here, in more detail, are steps to follow in making a survival still, and with an optional refinement added—a drinking tube that eliminates need for having to pull up the pail whenever you want to get at the water.

Pick an unshaded spot and dig the hole, using a stick or even your hands if you have no shovel. The hole

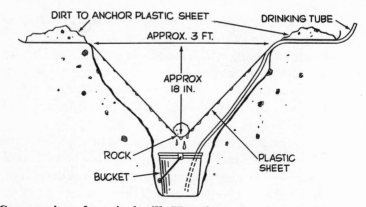

Cross section of survival still. Heat from the sun vaporizes ground water. The vapor condenses under the plastic, trickles down into bucket. Water can then be sucked up through tube. Still can produce up to 2 quarts of water a day. *Courtesy of D. S. Halacy, Jr.*

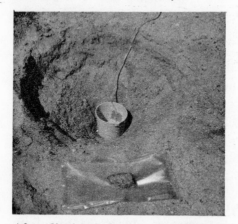

After digging hole, tape drinking tube to inside of bucket and set bucket at the bottom of the hole. Run the tube out of the hole and lay it on the ground.

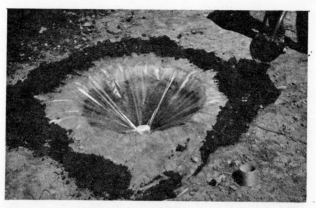

Lay plastic sheet over the hole, holding it in place with dirt stacked around the edges. Put a rock in the center of the plastic sheet and adjust the sheet so the rock is suspended a few inches above the bucket.

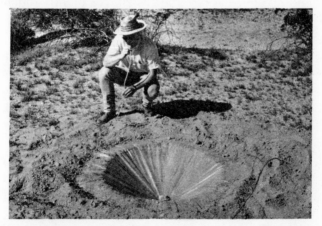

Water can be sucked up from bucket through the tube. Within twenty-four hours, still should yield a pint of water. Plastic-sheet cone also serves as a basin to catch water in case it rains.

should be about 36 inches in diameter at the top and for a few inches down, then should slope toward the bottom as the diagram shows. Dig deep enough so the point of the plastic cone can be about 18 inches below ground and still a couple of inches above the top of the bucket. The bucket can be 2- to 4-quart capacity. In a pinch, you can substitute a coffee can.

If you're going to use the drinking tube, which is optional, you need a 5-foot length of flexible plastic tubing. Tape one end inside the bucket or can and set the container at the bottom of the hole, centered. Bring the rest of the tube up and out of the hole.

Now lay the plastic sheet over the hole. Any clear plastic will work but especially good for the purpose is Tedlar plastic, an adherable material made by Dupont and marketed as No. 100 BG-20. It's slightly roughened and allows drops of water to cling more effectively than ordinary plastic.

Stack up dirt around the edge of the plastic—enough to hold it securely. Put a rock—about fist-size—in the center of the plastic sheet and then make any adjustments around the edges necessary to bring the rock and sheet center down to within a few inches of the top of the bucket.

Make certain the plastic cone doesn't touch earth anywhere. It's a help—but not absolutely critical—if you can manage to get 2 or 3 inches of air space between the inverted plastic cone and the earth.

You'll soon begin to see vapor form under the plastic and then drops begin to trickle down to the bucket. You won't be drinking water imediately but within twenty-four hours you should have at the very least a pint. It will be distilled water, of course, and will have a flattish taste—but the distillation makes it safe to drink.

If, by some happy chance, it should begin to rain, the inverted cone of your survival still will act as a catch basin and hold the water.

14   On the Water

Canoe camping is increasingly popular with outdoorsmen, many of whom now use outboard motors to travel
faster and further. Hundreds of thousands of others are
using everything from prams to de luxe small craft to
wander for weekends or longer with lightweight camping equipment aboard.

Float trips have their enthusiasts who find they may
produce more fish and pleasure than any other kind of
camping jaunt. Ordinarily, float trips are smooth trips—
but they've been known to get rough.

There are, in fact, always hazards on the water—
always some chance of landing *in* the water. And while
it helps to be a good swimmer, even expert swimmers
can get into trouble.

One of the most important preparations you can
make for any water jaunt is to learn the technique of
drownproofing if you don't already know it. It's not
difficult to learn nor to teach to children. Knowing the
technique, even a non-swimmer can stay afloat for
hours. And so can an injured person with a broken arm
or leg.

What Drownproofing Is

Essentially, it's a technique of floating that allows
anyone to handle emergencies in water without panic or

exhaustion—the causes of nearly all drownings. The big difference between a drownproofed swimmer and even an expert undrownproofed one is that the former doesn't get tired regardless of how long he is afloat or how far he has to swim.

Developed by Fred R. Lanoue, head swimming coach at Georgia Institute of Technology in Atlanta, the technique is taught by the U.S. Navy and all service academies as an important element of survival training, and has become part of the required curriculum for freshmen at more than a score of colleges. Drownproofing has been taught to more than 30,000 people in the Atlanta area.

Lanoue also has taught 350 physicians the technique with the hope that family doctors and pediatricians especially can help spread its use by bringing the technique to the attention of patients, school boards and other agencies concerned with health and safety.

In one notable experiment at Georgia Tech, Lanoue proved that crippled people unable to use their arms and legs could survive for long periods in deep water by his method.

He picked a group of poor swimmers, bound the ankles of twenty, bound the wrists and ankles of another twenty. All went into the water and bobbed around without sinking. Average time in the water for the group as a whole was four hours and forty-three minutes. Sixteen of those who took part in the experiment chose to stay afloat for a solid eight hours.

Not long ago, Lanoue lectured to a civic group in Atlanta. One of the members had a large swimming pool. Lanoue demonstrated the technique with a group of 4-year-old children. "All of the children," he says, "stayed afloat during the entire lecture—more than an hour—and most were able to do so with their hands and feet tied. Almost every member of that club has since been drownproofed."

According to Lanoue, 99½ percent of the human race will float on the surface of the water when the lungs are full of air. Yet, he says, "most drownings are caused by ignorance of the laws of floating bodies. A weak swimmer, finding himself beyond his depth with no help readily available, struggles until he is exhausted and then goes down. A strong swimmer, seized by cramps, gives way to terror and thrashes about wildly until he is too exhausted to save himself.

"The answer in both cases is this: don't struggle—take a deep breath and let yourself sink.

"You will come up again, close to the surface, and a gentle flip with your hands or legs will raise your head just enough above the water to allow you another breath. Then let yourself go and sink again.

"Don't fight, don't struggle. Just relax. Save your energy—and you will live."

The conventional method of floating on one's back, Lanoue points out, can be dangerous under certain conditions. "It's easy to swallow excessive amounts of water from waves that break over the head, and then the swimmer is in serious trouble."

The Steps to Follow

Lanoue breaks his system down into a series of simple steps.

1. Take a deep breath and with your lungs full of air, relax. Relax all over. Let your hands dangle and allow your face to fall forward in the water. Let yourself sink vertically in the water and just stay relaxed.

2. Get ready for a change of breath. As you practice, you'll be able to hold your breath longer and longer. But, in any case, take a fresh breath before you actually have to. To get ready, just leisurely cross your arms, keeping the forearms together. At the same time, raise one knee toward your chest and raise and extend the other foot behind you.

3. Now, without changing position of arms and legs, raise your head from its horizontal position to the vertical, quickly but smoothly, and stop with the bottom of your chin still in the water. Even as you begin to raise your head, start to exhale through the nose. Continue to exhale as your nose emerges from the water.

4. When you're finished exhaling, you're ready to inhale through the mouth. To keep your mouth above water for that, gently sweep the palms of your hands outward and step downward on the water with both feet, moving easily, with the minimum of effort. In fact, it's important that you don't move so vigorously that you pop your shoulders up out of the water. Inhale through your open mouth.

5. After you've inhaled, close your mouth and relax. Let your face drop down to horizontal position, allow your arms and legs to dangle, and sink vertically into the water. If you find that in a pool or in rough fresh water you tend to sink several feet below the surface, you can overcome the tendency with an easy downward stroke of arms and legs.

THE TECHNIQUE OF DROWNPROOFING

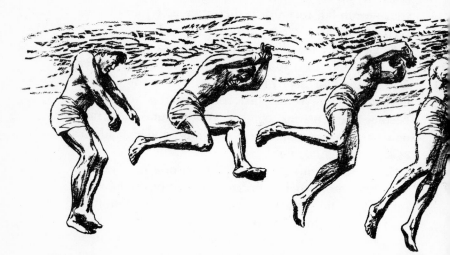

Take deep breath, relax. Let yourself sink in the water with face forward.

Ready to change breath. Cross arms, raise one knee, raise other foot behind you.

Raise head, start to exhale through nose. Continue to exhale as nose clears water.

Inhale through mouth, sweeping palms outward, stepping down with feet.

6. Now just rest, limply hanging in the water. When you feel you're ready to take another breath, go through steps 2 to 5 again.

The system takes a little practice but just about anybody who is willing to try can learn it quickly. There will be individual variations in three things: the amount of air to be exhaled, the amount to be inhaled, and the length of the rest period, step 6. With a little experimenting, you can establish what works best for

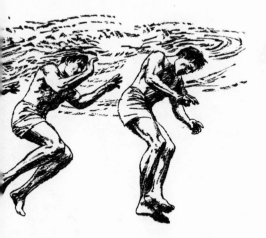

Close mouth, relax, let your face come forward, dangle arms. Sink.

Rest under the water, limply, until you need a breath. Then repeat sequence.

you. One thing to note: If your chest feels tight under water, it's a sign that you are either not exhaling enough or you are resting too long.

Drownproofed Traveling

With the basic technique outlined above, you can survive for hours in the water, staying afloat without tiring.

THE TECHNIQUE OF

| Inhale when head comes above water, just as in drownproofing system. | As head goes under water, tip it forward, opening legs and raising rear foot high. | Extend arms forward and upward, keeping the hands together. Scissors kick. | As feet close in kick, sweep arms outward and to the sides, bringing them to thighs. | As you glide forward, keep hands at sides and exhale through your nose. |

Lanoue has also developed a travel stroke that will allow you to propel yourself forward steadily for long periods, making it to shore if it's a mile or more away.

The travel stroke starts toward the end of the basic drownproofing sequence, after you've inhaled and begun to sink vertically.

As soon as your head goes below the water, tip it forward and at the same time open your legs, getting the rear foot as high as you can.

Next, extend your arms forward and upward, keeping the hands together.

As soon as your arms are fully extended, scissors-kick with your legs.

DROWNPROOFED TRAVELING

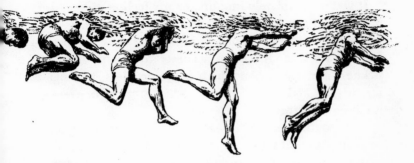

When you need air, bow your back, raise knees to chest to return to vertical.	Once vertical, cross arms in front of head to begin drownproof breathing method.	Inhale through mouth, sweeping palms outward and stepping downward with feet.	After you've taken a breath, allow yourself to sink and repeat travel sequence.

As your feet come together in the kick, slowly and easily sweep your arms outward and to the sides until they end up touching your thighs.

As the result of the kick and sweep, you'll glide forward and toward the surface. As you glide, keep your body relaxed and your hands at your thighs, and begin to exhale through your nose.

When you're ready for a fresh breath—without waiting until you actually feel the need—return to the vertical position by bowing your back and bringing your knees up toward your chest.

With your body in vertical position, you're ready to go into the basic drownproof sequence for changing breaths.

Motion Sickness

If you're completely immune to any feeling of queasiness aboard a boat, you're fortunate. Bad enough even when it's mild, seasickness can be a serious business when it's severe. It's more accurate to call it motion sickness—for it's motion which is the problem, whether it's the rise and roll of a boat, swaying of car or train, lurching of plane.

The trouble lies in unusual sensitivity of an inner ear structure, the labyrinth, a series of semicircular canals that provide balance. In the sensitive, they are overstimulated by motion and send out impulses that produce a series of symptoms.

Among the early symptoms are yawning, mild nausea, and a feeling of lassitude. The face becomes drawn, the color poor; the victim loses interest in his surroundings, may break out into a cold sweat. Hiccups also sometimes occur. Next comes vomiting; with that, generalized weakness often develops. When it's prolonged, severe motion sickness can lead to abnormal lowering of blood pressure, weight loss, dehydration, and depression.

Some people who develop motion sickness in mild degree are able to adapt after a time to the motion and feel well. But the adaptation often breaks down if the motion gets rougher or otherwise more extreme. Also, unhappily, the adaptation may last the trip but then disappear and have to be developed all over again on the next trip.

Many drugs are useful for countering motion sickness. If you're particularly sensitive, a doctor will be glad to prescribe one. Among the most effective are cyclizine,

50 milligrams by mouth before a trip, then 50 milligrams three times a day before meals; dimenhydrinate, in similar dosage; meclizine, 25 to 50 milligrams once a day; and promethazine, 25 milligrams twice a day.

Certain other measures are helpful for severe motion sickness when coupled with medication—and often help, without medication, when the sickness isn't severe.

Aboard a boat, stay above deck in the fresh air. Avoid alcohol. Until you feel better, take fluids and only the simplest of foods—in small amounts, at short intervals. Also, until you feel better, avoid reading, playing cards, or any activities that require close eye attention.

Car, Train and Plane Sickness

When you travel by car, you can often lessen mild discomfort by avoiding long intervals of driving, routinely stopping often. Stop, too, as soon as you feel any active nausea coming on; a brief stop then may get rid of the nausea quickly and allow you to proceed. Eat—but lightly and more often than usual. In a car, best position for avoiding motion sickness is the right front seat.

On a train, if you begin to feel sick, get up immediately, move about, stand on the platform or in the hall where air circulation is better. Avoid riding in the last couple of coaches on a train; they sway more.

On a plane, a seat in the center between the wings is the best position. If mild symptoms develop, hold your head as still as possible and close your eyes.

Part III

MEDICAL EMERGENCIES
AND FIRST AID

15   What to Pack

Even minor illnesses and injuries can spoil a trip if they cannot be promptly treated. A basic first-aid kit is very much worth taking along even for the simplest and shortest jaunt. Something more may be needed by the outdoorsman who moves far away from roads and telephones and cannot count on the quick arrival of medical help in case of a serious emergency.

Basic Kit

You can buy a standard basic first-aid kit or put together one of your own.

It should include the following items:

Triangular bandages, 40"; at least one, preferably 3 to 4, each with 2 safety pins. For bandaging over sterile dressings; for arm and hand sling; for pressure bandage for sprains and strains; for splinting broken bones; for use as a tourniquet when no other method controls severe bleeding.

Sterile first-aid dressing, 2" x 2", in sealed envelope. Box of 12. For small wounds.

Sterile first aid dressing, 4" x 4", in sealed envelope. Box of 12. For larger wounds and for compress to stop bleeding.

Roller bandage 1" x 5 yds., 2. For use as a finger bandage.

Roller bandage 2" x 5 yds., 2. To hold dressings in place.

Adhesive tape, 1 roll. To hold dressings in place.

Mild soap, 1 bar. For cleansing of wounds, scratches and cuts. Also to cleanse your hands before applying first aid to wounds. (If you wish, you can obtain antiseptic soap in plastic squeeze tubes with 2" gauze pads.)

Table salt and baking soda, 1 small package of each. For use in case of shock. Dissolve 1 teaspoon salt, ½ teaspoon baking soda in 1 quart water.

Scissors with blunt tips, 1 pair. For cutting bandages or clothing.

Tweezers, 1. To remove stingers from insect bites, splinters, thorns, etc.

Eye dropper, 1. For rinsing eyes.

Aspirin, box of 12 5-grain tablets. For headache and pain relief.

The above is a minimum list which should serve up to four people under ordinary conditions when you're not deep in the wilderness, far from medical help.

Note that an antiseptic is not included. The American Medical Association advises that antiseptics are not necessary for cleansing wounds, scratches and cuts; mild soap will do.

If you'd like nevertheless to have an antiseptic along,

the U.S. Department of Agriculture, which publishes a
manual for employees working in areas where medical
facilities are not readily available, advises povidone-
iodine complex.

Basic Kit—Some Additions to Consider

A thermometer.

Aromatic spirits of ammonia. For fainting.

Calamine lotion. For relieving itching from insect
bites and stings and poisonous plants.

Snake bite kit, suction type. If you're going into snake-
infested country, you may want to take one of these
along. Sporting goods and drug stores have such kits,
some of which take up little more room than a 12-gauge
shell.

Insect-sting kit. This is for emergency treatment if
you or anyone in your party is especially sensitive and
reacts extremely to bites of such insects as bees, wasps,
hornets, and yellow jackets. A new kit just marketed is
small enough to fit in a shirt pocket and contains a
sterile hypodermic syringe with epinephrine, a tourniquet, sterile alcohol pad, two 4-milligram chlorphenira-
mine maleate tablets, two phenobarbital-ephedrine tablets, and instructions. It's priced at $3.80, made by
Center Laboratories, Inc., Port Washington, N.Y. You
will need a doctor's prescription for it.

A Kit for Deep in the Wilderness

If you're going into a remote area where it may not
be possible to get medical help quickly when it's needed
during serious illnesses or injuries, it may be wise to add

a number of other items to those in your basic first aid kit.

Suturing Equipment

If you're far from a doctor, having along equipment for suturing or stitching up a wound—and knowing how to use it—can be of great value.

Here is what one physician, himself an enthusiastic outdoorman, advises, (and it would be highly desirable to check with your own physician for additional advice he can provide in greater detail and perhaps for some basic instruction he may be willing to give):

A sterile suture package is available with the nylon thread joined to the end of a needle. Size 3-0 is generally useful except for the face; 5-0, finer, is less likely to leave a scar.

The needle can be held with an instrument called a hemostat—a clamp that amounts to a small, self-locking, needle-nosed plier. It's also useful for extracting thorns, fishhooks, and even for repairs on fishing and other equipment.

Suturing may be needed only when a gaping wound cannot be held together any other way. In most cases, but not all, the edges of a wound can be pulled together and held by tape. Deep cuts in areas subject to much movement sometimes prove to be problems.

When suturing appears to be absolutely essential, first wash the wound with soap and water, then dry it.

Hold the needle with the clamp and take the stitch through the skin, never beyond that into fat or muscle. The skin is never more than a quarter of an inch thick.

If you stay within it, you penetrate no vital structure. There is some chance of hitting a blood vessel. In that case, pull the suture through and out and start again in another site just a little above or below. Bleeding will stop if you apply pressure for a minute or so.

Avoid suturing near an eyelid since the skin may be distorted during healing and cause trouble later.

There is some pain with suturing—but it's not agonizing and it lasts for just a second or two.

After taking the stitch, tie the thread. Cut the extra, leaving the stitch ends about $\frac{1}{4}$ inch long to help remove them in about seven days.

Special Drugs

You'll need prescriptions for these. They are potent drugs which should not be used indiscriminately. Your doctor almost certainly will oblige if you explain the purpose. There are alternate medications which can be used in place of those listed here and your physician may have suggestions about these along with additional information about when and how best to use them.

For eye injuries: A mixture of local anesthetic, antibiotic and anti-inflammatory agent. One such is a mixture of equal parts of Pontocaine and Neohydeltrasol (neomycin plus cortisone). A drop every three hours helps provide relief if the eye is hit by an object such as a flying wood chip. It also helps in relieving snow blindness.

For nausea and vomiting: One drug helpful in preventing and controlling nausea, vomiting and retching is Compazine.

For diarrhea: Paregoric is useful. It's liquid, however, and subject to spillage. One newer agent, Lomotil, is available in tablet form and is often prescribed for diarrhea associated with various gastrointestional troubles, including acute infections and food poisonings.

For major infections: Penicillin, a tetracycline or other antibiotic in capsule form. Your physician can prescribe a dozen or so—enough to help in a case of blood poisoning, pneumonia or other severe infection. He'll tell you how to use them properly.

16   Basic Principles
of First Aid

The first-aid instructions in the following pages apply to a wide variety of situations which the outdoorsman may encounter. They are based upon recommendations of the American National Red Cross, the American Medical Association, the Forest Service Guide and U.S. Department of Agriculture Guide, and those of experienced physicians.

How to Proceed in a Serious Emergency

Most accidents and illnesses on hunting, fishing and other outdoor trips are minor. The first aid to be used for them will be obvious.

In case of serious trouble, however, it can be vital to follow this sequence of action:

1. Examine the patient carefully—and keep calm. As much as a dressing or splint, the victim may need the steadying influence of your calmness. Along with physical distress, he may be in some mental and emotional distress even though he doesn't show it.

2. Treat immediately those injuries or effects which can cause quick death. Do these things first:

Restore breathing
Stop severe bleeding

Treat poisoning

Treat shock

The proper methods will be described later.

3. Send someone for help if you can. If that's not possible, signal. Three rifle shots in quick succession are commonly recognized as a distress signal and may bring help. If you build a smoky fire, it may be seen by a fire tower lookout.

4. Keep the victim lying down. Protect him from unnecessary movement and manipulation.

5. If you've given the urgent first aid—for bleeding, shock, etc.—and have attended to obvious injuries, and if you can expect the arrival of medical help shortly, you may not need to make any further examination. A cardinal rule is to do no more than necessary until professional help arrives. Keep the patient as comfortable as possible—with a sunshade if needed or a blanket or coat for warmth. If you suspect internal injuries, do not give anything to drink. Don't pour anything down the mouth of an unconscious or partly conscious person; it may enter the windpipe. If the victim is unconscious, loosen clothing about his neck; and if there is no fracture, turn him on his side so any secretions can drool out from the corner of his mouth.

NOTE: A serious emergency warrants every possible attempt to get professional help. And professional help may be available even under what seem like the most unlikely circumstances. Many doctors are enthusiastic outdoorsmen: there could be a physician hunting, fishing or setting up camp not far from you, just around the bend of a wilderness trail. Many wilderness areas today are served by rescue units with doctors who can parachute to the site of an accident or helicopters and trained personnel capable of safely moving the seriously injured or ill from wilderness to hospital in hours.

6. If you must move the victim even just a short distance before a doctor arrives, check carefully for all possible injuries before making the move so you can support them properly during transport.

In some cases, this is simple—when the nature of the emergency clearly indicates only a single exposed part of the body has been injured, or in a poisoning incident, for example, when there is hardly any possibility of fractures, lacerations, etc.

But in other cases—falls, gunshot wounds, blows— you have to consider the possibility of injuries at other than the obvious sites. Consider every part of the body— head, neck, arms, trunk, legs. Surface injuries will be easy to discover. With a fracture, there may or may not be any visible evidence; with an internal injury, there almost never is. Use caution in removing clothing, explore gently. If you have the slightest suspicion that there may be a fracture or other injury, keep that part of the body from twisting and bending.

17 Medical Emergencies and First Aid Guide

Heavy Bleeding

Severe bleeding comes from wounds to one or more large blood vessels. Heavy loss of blood can kill in 3 to 5 minutes, sometimes even less.

WASTE NO TIME.

TRY TO STOP THE BLEEDING AT ONCE, ALWAYS IF POSSIBLE WITH PRESSURE DIRECTLY OVER THE WOUND.

Use a pad—clean handkerchief, clean cloth, whatever is available instantly. If nothing else is, use an item of clothing. Rather than delay, use even your bare hand. Worry about infection later. The first objective must be to control the hemorrhaging and save life.

Press pad—or hand—directly over wound. Most external bleeding can be controlled by pressure. Once you have it under control, apply cloth material if you have used your hand to now. If you've already used cloth, apply additional layers to form a sizeable covering, then bandage firmly with cloth strips, neckties, etc.

Don't remove bandage. If blood saturates it, add more layers of cloth and tighten the whole dressing directly over wound.

Raise the bleeding part higher than the rest of the body if no bones are broken.

First step in control of heavy
bleeding is to apply pressure
with pad directly over wound.

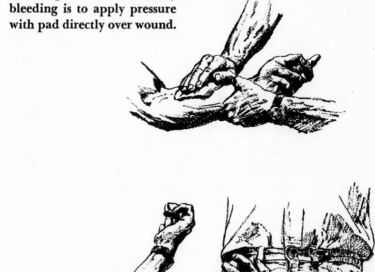

If direct pressure on wound does not stop heavy bleeding,
apply pressure with fingers at either of two main points.
Pressure on inner arm will stop bleeding below this point;
pressure with heel of hand just below groin will stop bleeding below this point.

If direct pressure on the wound fails to stop the flow, apply firm strong pressure to a pressure point where you can press the supplying blood vessel against underlying bone. This will reduce, though not necessarily completely stop, the bleeding.

There are two points on each side of the body where pressure may be of value:

1. On inner half of the arm, midway between elbow and armpit; pressure here will reduce bleeding in the arm below the pressure point.

2. Just below the groin on the front, inner half of the thigh; pressure here will reduce bleeding below.

Tourniquet

This is a last resort, needed only rarely, never to be used unless the bleeding seems certain to kill. Use of a tourniquet may save life but it involves a high risk of losing a limb. If it must be used, apply only a strong, wide piece of cloth—never a wire, rope or other narrow material. Wrap around upper part of limb, above wound; tie a half knot; put a short stick above the half knot; tie a full knot over the stick. Twist stick just tight enough to stop bleeding. Loosen for a few seconds every 15 minutes.

After bleeding has been controlled, keep the victim warm. If he is conscious and can swallow, give him liquids—water, tea, coffee but not alcoholic drinks. If he is unconscious or if abdominal injury is suspected, do not give fluids.

To apply a tourniquet, wrap a strong, wide cloth around limb above the wound. Tie half a square knot.

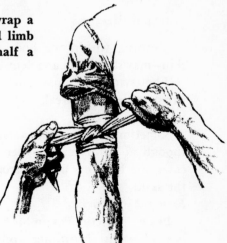

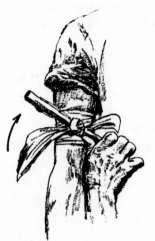

Place a short stick over the half knot and complete the knot over the stick. Twist stick to tighten.

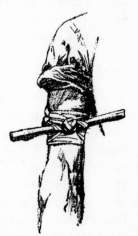

Secure the stick with the tails of the tourniquet. Be sure to loosen the tourniquet for a few seconds every 15 minutes.

Internal Bleeding

Bleeding within the body—without a break in the skin—may stem from a violent blow.

The symptoms may include restlessness, anxiety, thirst, pale face, weak and rapid pulse, generalized weakness.

Sometimes blood may come from mouth or nose though no injury can be seen in these organs. In such cases, the bleeding may be from lungs, stomach, within the skull.

First-aid treatment

Place the victim flat on his back. EXCEPTION: If he has difficulty breathing, pillow up his head and shoulders.

Keep him quiet and as reassured as you can.

Try to have him control vomiting movements. Turn his head to the side for vomiting.

Do not give stimulants even if bleeding stops.

Move him only in flat-on-back or slightly propped position to a hospital.

Nosebleed

Nosebleeds may follow injury or occur spontaneously and are often more annoying than serious. Occasionally, however, the bleeding is heavy, prolonged and dangerous.

First-aid treatment

Have victim remain quiet, seated with head back, breathing through mouth.

Pinch nostrils together. Maintain the pinching pressure for 5 to 10 minutes.

Cold wet towels applied to face often help.

If bleeding fails to stop, pack gauze into nostril from which blood is coming, then pinch.

To Restore Breathing

Normal breathing may stop as the result of drowning, smoke inhalation, gas poisoning, electric shock, choking, poisoning by barbiturates and other drugs that depress respiration.

In most cases, death will follow within 6 minutes unless artificial respiration is given.

Artificial respiration may be needed, too, when breathing movements do not stop entirely but become slow and shallow or when lips, tongue and fingernails become blue. When in doubt, start artificial respiration; it cannot harm, may be lifesaving.

Seconds count. Do not stop to move victim unless absolutely essential because of dangerous conditions. Do not stop to look for help, loosen clothing or apply stimulants.

Begin immediately after checking mouth for obstructions and removing, if necessary, any foreign objects.

Mouth-to-Mouth Method

Place victim on his back if possible.

Put one hand under his neck and lift. With other hand holding top of his head, tilt head back.

Keep in place the hand that holds top of head. With the other that was under the neck, pull the victim's chin up to get a free air passage.

Take a deep breath and place your mouth over the

MOUTH-TO-MOUTH RESUSCITATION FOR ADULTS

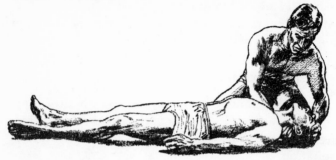

Lift victim's neck with one hand and tilt the head back by holding top of the head with other hand.

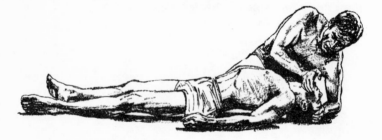

Pull victim's chin up with the hand that was lifting the neck. This insures a free air passage.

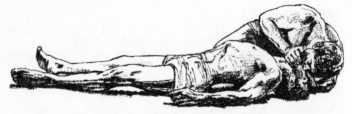

Take a deep breath, place your mouth over victim's mouth and pinch his nostrils. Breathe into victim's lungs until you see his chest rise. Remove your mouth and let him exhale. Repeat this cycle as rapidly as victim's lungs empty themselves for first few minutes, then 15 times per minute.

MOUTH-TO-MOUTH RESUSCITATION FOR INFANT OR SMALL CHILD

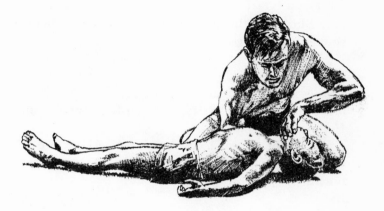

Lift victim's neck with your right hand and with your left lift his lower jaw so that it juts out.

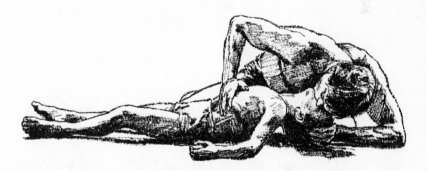

Place your mouth over the victim's *mouth and nose,* making a leakproof seal, and breath into his lungs gently until you see the chest rise and you feel the lungs expand.

victim's mouth, making a leakproof seal. Pinch his nostrils to close them off.

NOW:

1. Blow your breath into the victim's mouth until you see his chest rise.

2. Remove your mouth and let the victim exhale while you take another breath.

Repeat the 2-step procedure—as rapidly as the victim's lungs empty themselves for the first few minutes, then 15 times per minute.

For infant or small child, use same procedure but with your mouth placed over the child's mouth and nose. Blow your breath in gently until you see the chest rise.

MANUAL METHOD

If for any reason you cannot use the mouth-to-mouth method, employ the manual method:

Place victim on back, face up, with something under his shoulders to raise them and allow the head to drop backward.

Kneel above the victim's head, facing him.

Grasp his wrists, cross them, and press them against his lower chest.

Immediately, pull his arms up, out and as far back as possible.

Repeat 15 times a minute.

If a second person is available to assist, have him hold the victim's head so it tilts backward and the jaw juts forward.

MANUAL METHOD OF RESUSCITATION

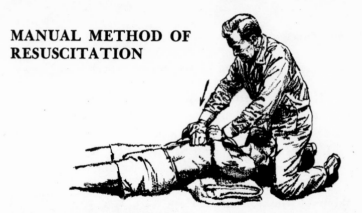

With the victim on his back, put something under his shoulders to raise them and allow head to drop backwards. Kneel at victim's head and grasp his arms at the wrists, crossing and pressing his wrists against the lower chest.

Immediately pull arms upward and outward as far as possible. Repeat this sequence 15 times a minute.

If a second rescuer is present, he should hold the victim's head so it tilts backward and the jaw juts forward.

ADVANTAGES OF MOUTH-TO-MOUTH METHOD

Mouth-to-mouth artificial respiration has a number of advantages, the American Medical Association points out.

If necessary, it can be used when the victim is in water or in cramped surroundings and cannot be placed on the ground. A rescuer can maintain the breathing for hours without fatigue. Hands are free to keep head tilted backward and jaw jutting forward, which prevents obstruction of the air passage, the most common cause of failure of artificial respiration. Also, the rescuer can see, feel and hear the effect of each lung inflation and can control the amount, rate and pressure of air administered to the victim.

HOW LONG TO CONTINUE

In many cases, the victim will start to breathe for himself within a few minutes after artificial respiration has been started.

But recovery often may be delayed in electric shock and drug and gas poisoning cases. In such cases, gas may have displaced oxygen in the blood stream or nerves and muscles involved in breathing may be paralyzed or deeply depressed. Artificial respiration then may have to be carried on for long periods.

If any case, continue artificial respiration until the victim begins to breathe for himself, or a physician pronounces him dead, or until he appears dead beyond any doubt.

See also the following.

Stopped Heart

If an injured person does not respond to artificial respiration, it may be because his heart is no longer beating. The heart is fairly certain to have stopped if you can feel no pulse at the wrist and hear no sound with your ear held to the victim's chest.

The following closed heart massage procedure may save a life if used promptly.

1. With victim on his back, raise legs to drain blood toward heart and support shoulders so neck is arched backwards.

2. Put the heel of one hand on the lower end of the breastbone and the other hand right on top of the first hand.

3. Press down firmly with both hands, then take both

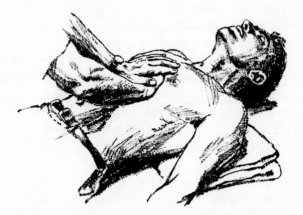

If a victim does not respond to artificial respiration, and you cannot feel his pulse or hear his heart, apply the closed heart massage.

hands away to allow the chest to expand. **Repeat every second.**

4. If you're the only rescuer present, stop every 30 seconds to use mouth-to-mouth artificial respiration 3 or 4 times. If another rescuer is present, have him do the mouth-to-mouth breathing once for every 5 repetitions of the heart massage you perform.

From time to time, check the pulse. In some cases, it will take only a few seconds before the heart starts to beat again.

Choking

When a foreign body—a chunk of food or anything else—lodges in the throat or air passages and causes choking, the urgent need is to get it out. If the victim still has difficulty breathing afterward, begin mouth-to-mouth artificial respiration.

To remove foreign bodies:

For adult: Place on side so head is lower than trunk— or have victim lean over back of a chair. Give him a sharp slap between shoulder blades. Clear his throat quickly with your fingers and pull his tongue forward.

For a small child: Hold, head down, over your arm or leg. Apply several sharp pats between shoulder blades. Clear throat quickly with fingers and pull tongue forward.

For an infant: Hold by ankles, allowing head to hang straight down. Open his mouth, pull tongue forward, let object fall out.

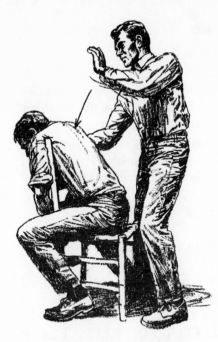

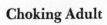

Choking Adult

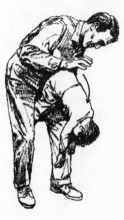

Choking Child

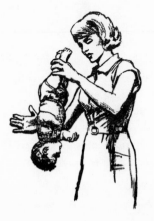

Choking Infant

Shock

Medical shock—totally unrelated to electric shock—can cause death from injuries and illnesses that in themselves would not be fatal.

Shock is a depressed body state caused by an upset of the delicate mechanisms which keep blood circulating regularly to all parts of the body. Because of the failure in circulation, the brain and other vital organs do not get the amount of blood needed to maintain life.

Some degree of shock may result from practically all except the most minor injuries. Shock may also follow infection, pain, disturbance of circulation by bleeding, stroke, heart attack, heat exhaustion, severe burns, food or chemical poisoning, broken bones and exposure.

IN EVERY HEALTH EMERGENCY, THINK OF SHOCK AND TAKE STEPS TO PREVENT AND COMBAT IT.

What to look for

Paling of the face.

Cold, clammy skin with drops of sweat on forehead and palms of hands.

Shallow, irregular breathing.

Trembling, nervousness, apprehension.

Nausea or vomiting.

Pulse weak, irregular, rapid.

Unconsciousness.

Note: Symptoms usually develop gradually, may not be readily apparent at first. Even if none is present in a severely injured person, the danger of shock is still real and it is advisable to carry out the following measures.

What to do

Keep the victim lying down—if possible, with his head lower than the rest of his body.

Raise his legs 12 to 18 inches if there are no broken bones.

Keep him warm if the weather is cold or damp. Cover him and conserve body heat with a blanket underneath. DON'T OVERHEAT. Keep him only warm enough to prevent shivering.

If the victim is conscious and able to swallow, give fluids. Shock solution often helps prevent or delay the appearance of shock. Make it by adding 1 teaspoon salt and ½ teaspoon baking soda (sodium bicarbonate) to 1 quart of water. Give as much of this solution as the victim is willing to take. If shock solution is not available, use water, tea, coffee—but not alcoholic beverages.

Caution: Do not give fluids if the victim is unconscious or semiconscious, if he is vomiting repeatedly, or if an abdominal injury is suspected.

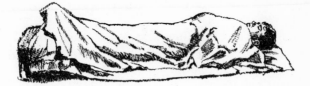

Treatment for Shock

Poisoning by Mouth

If the victim is unconscious or otherwise unable to explain, suspect poisoning from one or more of the following:

Odor of poison on the breath.

Discoloration of lips and mouth.

Confusion or sudden illness.

Telltale container.

What to do

Speed is essential. The objective is to act if possible before the body has time to begin absorbing the poison or, at least, before it has absorbed all of it.

If antidote is known (labels on containers of potentially poisonous materials indicate antidotes)—and if it is available—give it.

Otherwise, DILUTE the poison with milk or water. Give four or more glasses.

If possible, even as one person is beginning treatment, another should try to call a physician or hospital.

Induce vomiting—*but only under certain circumstances.*

DO NOT induce it if victim—

is unconscious;

has pain and burning sensation in mouth or throat;

is known to have swallowed any petroleum product (kerosene, gasoline, lighter fluid);

is known to have swallowed an acid (nitric, acetic, hydrochloric, etc.);

is known to have swallowed an alkali (lye or caustic soda, potash, strong ammonia water).

DO induce vomiting in other cases. Induce it by

placing your finger at the back of the victim's throat—or by administering a glass of warm water containing two tablespoons of salt.

When retching and vomiting start, place the victim face down, head lower than hips, to prevent vomitus from getting into the lungs and causing additional damage. If the poison is unknown, save the vomitus for examination by a physician.

Poisoning—Skin Contamination

Drench the affected skin area with water.

Apply more water—a stream of it—on the skin while removing any clothing covering the area.

And cleanse the skin thoroughly again with more water.

The quicker and more thoroughly you can dilute and wash away the poison, the less the extent of injury.

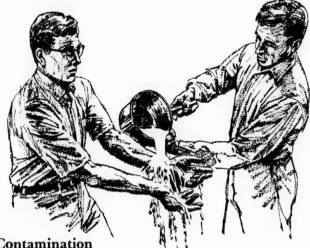

Skin Contamination

Poisoning—Snake Bites

Snake bites cause no more than ten to twenty deaths annually in the United States. Of poisonous bites, about 2 percent prove fatal.

There are four kinds of poisonous snakes in this country. Three—rattlesnakes, copperheads and cotton-mouth moccasins—are pit vipers. The fourth—the coral snake—belongs to the cobra family.

The pit vipers have a small, deep pit or depression between the eyes and nostrils, giving them the appearance of having an extra set of nostrils. They grow quite large, particularly the rattlers, which cause most snake-bite fatalities.

Coral snakes are small, have brilliant markings: broad red and black bands separated by narrow bands of yellow.

Except for the coral snake, which chews rather than bites, poisonous snakes leave typical fang punctures. Nonpoisonous types leave two U-shaped rows of tooth marks. With a nonvenomous snake bite, there is little pain, and swelling is no greater than usual for any wound.

Poison bite symptoms

These may include general weakness, shortness of breath, nausea and vomiting, weak and rapid pulse, dimming of vision, faintness progressing to unconsciousness.

What to do

Have the victim lie down and stay as quiet as possible. Moving increases the rate of poison absorption.

Tie a constricting band above the bite. It should be

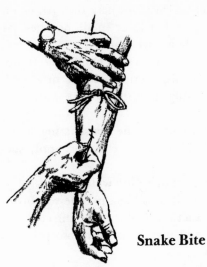
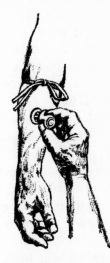

Snake Bite

tight enough to make surface veins stand out but not tight enough to shut off blood flow in deeper blood vessels. Loosen every 15 minutes for a few seconds.

Begin immediately to remove as much venom as possible from the wound by a combination of skin cuts and suction—this way:

Sterilize a knife or razor blade with a match flame. Make crosscuts, about 1/4-inch long and about that deep, through fang marks. *Caution:* Be careful not to cut too deeply and injure muscles and nerves, especially in hand and wrist, where they lie immediately below the skin.

Apply suction to the cuts to remove as much venom from the bite as possible. Use a suction cup if available—or your mouth. Venom is not a stomach poison but it is advisable to rinse the fluid from the mouth.

Continue suction for at least an hour. If you have no suction cup, lips and cheek muscles may tire. An emergency measure is to heat a bottle or small-mouthed jar with hot water (or burn a piece of paper in it, and apply it immediately over the cuts. Don't get it hot enough to burn. As it cools, suction will be produced. Reheat·and reapply, using mouth suction while the bottle is being reheated.

If the swelling spreads up to the constricting band, move the band higher. Make more cuts and apply suction.

Give the patient plenty of drinking water.

Apply cold water or ice if possible any time you break off briefly from using suction. Cold at the affected site gives some pain relief and may help slow absorption of poison into the system.

Get medical help. If it's necessary to transport the victim to doctor or hospital, keep the injured part lower than the rest of the body and continue to apply cold compresses to it.

Poisoning—Black Widow Spider and Scorpion Bites

Symptoms may include slight swelling and redness at the bite site; local pain which may begin to spread throughout the body; profuse sweating; nausea; painful cramps of abdominal and other mucles.

What to do

Keep the victim lying quietly and warm.

Apply a constricting band above the bite, loosening it every 15 minutes.

Apply cold compresses over bite.

Get medical attention. Almost all victims of black widow spider and scorpion bites recover. Death occurs only occasionally in infants and young children and may conceivably occur in older, infirm people. Nevertheless, the course of illness for a day or more may be stormy and a physician can use helpful measures against pain and systemic symptoms.

Abscess

An abscess is a collection of pus, usually the result of an infection. It is part of the body's protective mechanism through which it tries to localize the infection, prevent its spread, and finally destroy or throw off the infecting organisms. When the abscess is near the surface, the affected area is usually hot, swollen, painful.

What to do

Rest the infected area.

If medical aid is not readily available, apply hot, wet dressings.

Appendicitis

Typically starts with pain in the navel region commonly accompanied by loss of appetite, nausea and vomiting, but usually not by diarrhea. After several hours, pain shifts to the lower right part of the abdomen and is continuous, accentuated by coughing, sneezing or jarring. There may be mild fever, 99 to 102 F.

What to do

Put the patient to bed.

Give no food, only sips of water.

Give no laxatives which may cause a rupture of the infected appendix and spread infection throughout the abdomen.

Get medical help as soon as possible.

Blisters

In general, if a blister can be protected against breaking, leave it alone. The fluid will be gradually absorbed by deeper layers of skin and the skin will soon return to normal.

If the blister is large or in a spot where it is likely to be broken, follow these steps:

Gently clean blister and area around it with soap and water.

Sterilize a needle over a flame and use it to puncture edge of blister.

Gently press edges of blister opposite point of puncture to force out the fluid slowly.

Apply a sterile gauze pad and adhesive.

If a blister has already broken, wash off the area carefully with soap and water and apply sterile gauze pad and adhesive.

Blisters

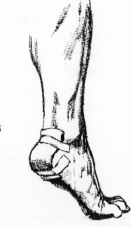

Boils

A round, reddened, painful, pea-like elevation, a boil is essentially dead tissue with pus containing millions of germs. Like an abscess, it's part of the body's protective mechanism—nature's effort to wall off an infection from surrounding tissue and keep it localized.

Don't squeeze. This will break the protective wall and cause spread of the infection.

If the boil is painful or shows signs of spreading, hot wet dressings may lessen the pain and hasten the coming-to-a-head process.

When the boil comes to a head and discharges, don't touch any of the pus. Wipe off promptly with a sterilized gauze to prevent contamination of skin about the boil. Cover with a sterile dressing.

Bruises

A bruise or contusion develops when a blow or fall breaks small blood vessels beneath the skin. It's the most common of all injuries. As blood oozes out of broken vessels into tissues under the skin, discoloration and painful swelling follow. Discoloration, at first reddish, soon changes to dark blue or purple, later to a brownish and then yellowish hue, and gradually fades as healing occurs.

What to do

In minor bruises, no first aid may be needed. For more severe ones, ice packs or cold cloths help reduce swelling and relieve pain. Bruises of an arm or leg will be less painful if the limb is elevated.

Burns

Burns are divided into three classes or degrees:

First degree—skin reddened but no damage to deeper layers.

Second degree—skin blistered because of injury to deeper skin layers but no damage to structures beneath.

Third degree—skin looks cooked or charred with damage to underlying tissues.

In addition to degree, the amount of body burned determines the seriousness of a burn. For example, a second-degree burn covering a large area such as the chest is likely to be more serious than a third-degree burn involving just a finger.

Shock is present in nearly every extensive burn and must be considered in all but the most minor burns.

Anybody with one-fourth of the body surface burned can develop such serious "burn shock" that he may die unless given immediate first aid. (About 18 percent of body surface would be represented by the equivalent of any of the following: all of one leg; all of one arm and the head; the front of the trunk; or the back of the trunk.)

Primary objectives of first aid are to control pain, combat shock, prevent infection.

What to do

For small first- and second-degree burns:

If skin is not broken, immerse burned part in clean, cold water or apply clean ice. This lessens pain, sometimes may even greatly shorten the course of the recovery from the burn.

Soak a sterile gauze pad or clean cloth in a baking soda solution, using 2 tablespoons of baking soda (sodium bicarbonate) to a quart of lukewarm water.

Apply wet pad to burn and bandage loosely.

For widespread second and third degree burns:

If you can get the victim quickly to doctor or hospital: Cover with sterile or clean dressing, treat for shock, and rush to medical help.

If you're in an isolated area:

1. Remove clothing from burn, just cutting around any cloth that may adhere to burned area and leaving it there.

2. Do not put oil, grease, ointments, antiseptics or any other substance on a serious burn. Cover the area completely with sterile dressing. Cover the dressing with 8 to 10 layers of loose sterile or clean dressing. Then bandage in place. Do not put the bandage on so tightly that it cuts off circulation—but do make it snug enough to protect the burned area from the air.

3. Treat for shock. (See SHOCK.)

4. Let the victim drink all he can of the shock solution (1 teaspoon salt and ½ teaspoon of baking soda in 1 quart of water).

5. Notify doctor that plasma may be needed.

6. DO NOT touch burn with fingers, breathe on it, break or drain blisters, or change the dressing—a doctor's job.

Chemical Burns

Immediately flush with water. This is the very first vital step. Flushing away the chemical quickly can greatly reduce the extent of injury and lessen the pain.

Keep applying a stream of water while removing clothing.

Then treat like any other burn.

For a chemical burn of an eye, do this:

Flush with water immediately. One effective way: Have the victim lie down, with head tilted slightly outward, and gently pour water into his eye from cup, pitcher or other container. Pour into the inner corner (nearest the nose) of the eye so it flows across the eye and out at the outer edge, not getting into the unaffected eye.

Cover the eye with a sterile compress, bandage in place, and get the victim to a physician as quickly as you possibly can.

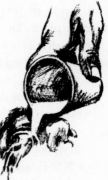

Chemical Burn in Eye

Sunburn

For mild cases, petrolatum, olive oil or cold cream may be soothing. So, too, calamine lotion.

If the burn is severe, treat as other burns.

Cold Exposure

After long exposure to excessive cold, the victim becomes numb, movement is difficult. Irresistible drowsiness may develop, his eyesight fails, and he may stagger and fall unconscious.

What to do

Get the victim into a warm room if possible—quickly.

Use artificial respiration if breathing has stopped.

Re-warm him as quickly as possible by wrapping in warm blankets.

When he responds, give him hot drinks.

Cuts and Abrasions

For minor wounds such as small cuts and abrasions (rubbing or scraping off of skin), it's important to prevent infection.

What to do

Immediately cleanse cut or abrasion and surrounding skin with soap and warm water. No antiseptic is needed. Avoid breathing on the wound or allowing fingers, used handkerchiefs, or other soiled material to touch it.

If there is bleeding, hold a sterile pad firmly over the wound until the bleeding stops. Then apply a fresh pad and bandage loosely with a triangular or roller bandage.

Dislocations

In a dislocation, the end of a bone is displaced from its normal position in the joint. The surrounding ligaments suffer some injury.

Dislocations may be the result of a fall, a blow against

a joint, a sudden twisting of the joint, or a sudden muscle contraction. Fingers, thumb and shoulder are most often affected.

Symptoms may include severe pain, swelling, loss of movement.

Unless properly relocated and cared for, a dislocation may recur repeatedly and cause disability.

What to do

Putting a serious dislocation back into place is a doctor's job. All dislocations should be handled according to the first-aid principles for fractures (See FRACTURES.)

The dislocated part should be kept quiet and medical attention obtained. Apply cold compresses and transport to doctor. Support a dislocated elbow or shoulder in a loose sling so it is kept immobilized during transport. If a hip is dislocated, move the victim on a wide board or stretcher made rigid. Use a pad of blankets or clothing large enough to support the leg on the injured side in the position the victim holds it.

Sometimes, in case of a dislocated finger, when medical facilities are far off, gentle traction may be tried. Pull cautiously—very cautiously—on the finger to try to bring the bone into place. If unsuccessful, do not persist. And do not attempt this on a dislocated thumb since there are more difficulties in the way and more risk of added injury.

Earache

Most often this is the result of an infection and should have medical attention even if first-aid measures provide some relief.

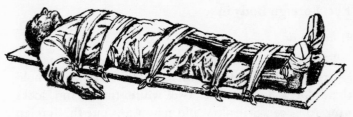

Dislocated Hip

Dislocated Finger

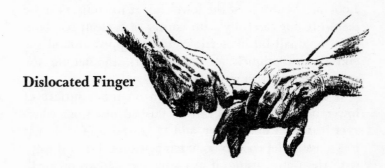

What to do

Heat or cold may help relieve pain—and there is no certain way to forecast in advance which may be more effective.

Try cold first—an ice bag or cold compress. If it doesn't provide adequate relief, switch to hot water bottle or hot compress.

If relief is still not adequate, a few drops of warm mineral oil in the ear may help.

Caution victim against blowing nose hard; this may aggravate the pain and infection.

Eye, Foreign Body in

What to do

Wash hands before touching the eye.

Bring upper eyelid down over the lower and hold there for a moment or two while the victim looks upward. Tears will flow and may wash out the foreign body.

If this fails to remove the object, carefully place your index and middle fingers just below the lower eyelid and use them to gently pull down on the lower lid. Look on the inside of the lower lid. If the object can be seen, lift out carefully with corner of a clean handkerchief or small bit of sterile cotton wrapped around the end of a toothpick (or equivalent), moistening the cotton slightly with water first.

If no foreign body can be seen on inner surface of lower lid, it sometimes can be flushed out from wherever it is. Boil some water, add 1/4 teaspoon of table salt to a glassful, let cool to body temperature. Flush the eye with the water, using, if available, an eyecup or medicine dropper.

Fainting

Among many possible causes of fainting are hunger, overfatigue, poor ventilation, standing for a long time, the sight of blood, and emotional upset.

Often a faint is preceded by paling of the face, sweating, drooping of the eyelids, and feelings of dizziness. At this point, a falling faint may be avoided if you get the victim to lie down or sit down with head between knees.

Once unconsciousness occurs, keep the victim lying

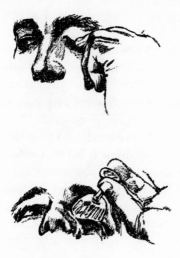

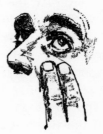

Foreign Body in Eye

down, with head lower than body. Loosen clothing. Sprinkling cold water on the victim's face or having him inhale aromatic spirits of ammonia often will help to restore consciousness.

Keep the victim resting quietly until he is fully recovered.

Fever

Fever, like pain, is a warning signal of something gone wrong. While there are many possible causes for temperature elevation, the most common is infection.
What to do

Get the victim to bed. Take his temperature.

Actually, fever is believed to be part of the body's

defense mechanism against infection. The trouble is that the body sometimes goes to extremes and a very high fever—in the neighborhood of 105° or 106°—may become a danger in itself. Until a doctor can be reached, you can use these measures to bring down excessive temperature:

Sponge with cool or tepid water. Sponge one part of the body at a time, keeping the remainder covered.

Apply ice bag or cold cloths to the head.

If the victim is conscious and there is no abdominal injury, give cold water by mouth.

If no doctor is available and you are carrying an antibiotic prescribed by your physician back home, follow his directions for using it in case of serious infection.

Fishhook Accidents

It's best, of course, to have the injured person seen by a physician. But this isn't always possible. First-aid care may be all that is available for some time.

What to do

If the hook is small or medium-sized, has penetrated only a little way (up to the barb or slightly past it), and

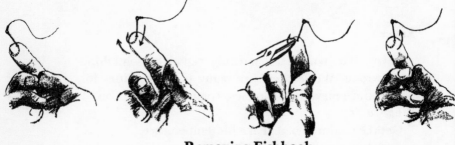

Removing Fishhook

if it is not in a critical area such as eye or face, a quick jerk may be the best way to remove it.

If the hook has penetrated deeper, past the barb, and is not in a critical area, the best method of removal may be to push it on through until the barb is free, then snip off the hook at the shaft and remove the two pieces.

After either of these maneuvers, if there has been very little bleeding, encourage some temporary blood flow as a help in eliminating any infectious organisms, particularly tetanus, by gentle pressure about the wound. Don't squeeze hard. Then apply a protective sterile dressing. Seek medical attention as soon as possible.

If the hook is large and has produced considerable damage, or if it is in a critical area about the face or eye, it's best not to try to remove it. Cover wound and hook with sterile dressing and get the victim to a doctor.

Foot Swelling

No uncommon problem on the trail, this is best relieved by removing shoes and socks, lying down, and propping the feet up. A wet cloth or towel wrapped around the bare feet will add to relief.

Fractures

A fracture is a broken bone. There are two kinds:
Closed—the bone is broken but the skin is intact.
Open (*Compound*)—the skin as well as bone is broken.

It is not always easy to determine whether there has been a break. It is probably a fracture when there is:

1. Tenderness over the injury with pain on movement.
2. Loss of ability to move the injured part.
3. Swelling and change in skin color.
4. Deformity.

But all of these signs may not be present. If you have any doubt about whether there has been a fracture or not, it's safest to treat the injury as a fracture.

Handle the patient gently. Rough or careless handling not only increases pain; it may also increase severity of shock, and cause broken bone ends to cut through muscle, nerves, blood vessels and skin.

Wherever the fracture may be, never try to set it yourself. Your objectives in first aid are to prevent further injury and counter shock until medical attention is available.

ARM OR LEG FRACTURE

If a physician is near, do not move either the limb or the patient.

What to do

If there is bleeding, cut away clothing and apply a pressure dressing. Place pad—sterile compress or clean handkerchief or cloth—over wound and press firmly directly over wound. Hold pad in place with strong bandage—neckties, cloth strips, etc.

If the victim must be moved, place the limb in as natural a position as possible without causing discomfort and apply splints. Splints must be long enough to extend beyond the joints above and below the fracture. You can use any firm material: board, pole, metal rod,

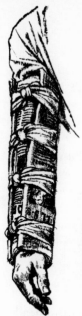

Fractured Arm

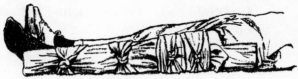

Fractured Leg

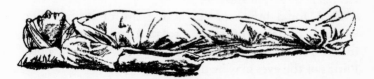

Fractured Skull

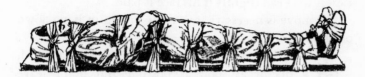

Neck or Back Fracture

even thick folded newspaper. Pad the splints with clothing or other soft material. Fasten splints with bandage or cloth at a minimum of three places: at the level of the break, at a point above the joint above the break, and at a point below the joint below the break.

Once splints are in place, check every 15–20 minutes to make certain swelling of the limb has not cut off circulation. Loosen splint bindings as necessary to deal with swelling.

Apply cold packs over the fracture and get the victim to a doctor or hospital.

Skull Fracture and Concussion

The most serious result of a fall or blow on the head is brain injury. Chief reason for concern in skull fracture is not so much the bone itself as the tissues beneath it. Brain injury or concussion can occur whether there has been an actual fracture or not.

Look for a bump or cut at the site of injury. The victim may be unconscious, or dazed and mentally confused. There may be bleeding from ears, mouth, nose. Pupils of the eyes may be different in size.

What to do

Keep the victim lying down. Prop up his head and shoulders if his face is either normal in color or flushed. Lower his head slightly if his face is pale.

If a move is necessary, move the victim in lying-down position.

Apply sterile gauze and bandage to open scalp wound.

Get a doctor as soon as possible but don't leave patient alone. Keep alert, ready if the victim should start choking on blood to lower his head and turn it carefully to drain.

NECK AND BACK FRACTURES

A symptom is pain in the neck or the spine.

The neck may be broken if the victim is not readily able to open and close his fingers or grip your hand firmly. If his fingers work but he cannot move feet or toes, the back may be broken.

If the victim is unconscious and you suspect spinal injury, treat as if the neck were fractured.

What to do

Don't let the victim move his head.

Cover with blankets.

Watch his breathing—and be ready to start mouth-to-mouth resuscitation if necessary (without moving his head).

Get a doctor or ambulance. The victim should not be moved unless there is no chance of getting medical help at the scene.

If a move must be made, it must be done with utmost caution. A twist or bend of broken neck or spine can kill. Take extreme care to avoid moving neck or spine while loading him on to rigid stretcher, board or poles.

Pad head well at sides to prevent motion. Tie hands across chest and tie head and body rigidly to board. Pad under the neck.

PELVIS FRACTURE

The pelvis—a basin-shaped bony structure extending outward from base of spine and curving toward the front of the body—provides a connection between spine and legs. It also protects many important organs and blood vessels lying in the lower part of the abdomen. Because these organs and vessels may be seriously damaged by broken bone ends, a pelvis fracture is a grave injury, requiring careful handling.

A symptom may be severe pain in the pelvis region while standing or walking; the pain may diminish or disappear while lying down. If there has been damage to organs or blood vessels, there may be difficulty in urinating or blood in the urine.

If you're not certain but have any reason to suspect a fracture after an injury to the pelvis region, treat as a fracture.

What to do

Combat shock (See SHOCK) which may be severe.

Bandage knees and ankles together. Keep the victim lying down. He will probably be most comfortable on his back with knees straight but let him bend knees if he wishes.

If he must be moved before he can receive medical aid, transport on back on rigid stretcher or board.

RIB FRACTURE

There is usually pain at the point of the break. Breathing is shallow since taking a deep breath—or coughing—increases pain. The point of fracture sometimes can be felt by running fingers gently along the rib. If the lung has been damaged by a broken rib bone, frothy or bright red blood may be coughed up.

What to do

If the broken rib has penetrated the skin and air is

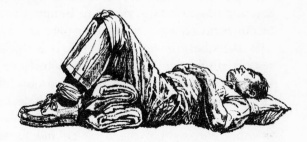

Pelvis Fracture

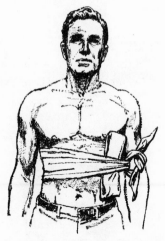

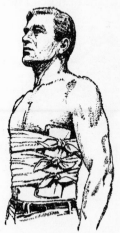

Rib Fracture

blowing in and out of the wound, apply an airtight dressing only. Get the victim to lie quietly. If he must be moved to a doctor, move him lying down.

If the chest is not punctured, tightly bandage to restrict rib motion. To do so, first loosely tie a triangular bandage or other broad bandage around the body at chest level so the knot will be on the side opposite the break. Put a folded cloth under the knot. As the victim breathes out, tighten the bandage and tie snugly. Repeat with two more bandages in the same way so they overlap slightly and cover the site of the fracture and adjacent areas.

Nose Fracture

Look for pain and tenderness in and about the nose; swelling and discoloration; possibly a change in usual shape of nose. There may be bleeding from the nose.

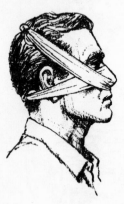

Nose Fracture

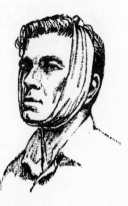

Jaw Fracture

What to do

If there is bleeding, hold lower end of nose between thumb and index finger and firmly press sides of nose against middle partition or septum for 4 or 5 minutes. Release pressure gradually. Apply cold cloths over nose. Have victim sit up, hold his head back slightly, and breathe through mouth.

Do not splint.

If there is a wound on the nose, apply a compress or protective dressing and fix in place with adhesive tape or bandage.

Get to doctor as soon as possible.

JAW FRACTURE

Look for pain on movement, inability to close the jaw properly. Teeth do not line up correctly. There is difficulty in speaking, drinking, swallowing.

What to do

Raise jaw gently with palm of your hand to bring lower and upper teeth together.

Put a bandage under chin and tie ends over top of head to support the jaw.

Remove bandage immediately if victim starts to vomit. Support jaw with hand. Rebandage when vomiting stops.

COLLARBONE FRACTURE

Severe pain and swelling may occur at site of break which sometimes can be found by gently running fingers over the area. The shoulder on the injured side will often be lower than the other since the collarbone is necessary for supporting the shoulder. Usually, the victim will be unable to raise his arm above the shoulder.

What to do

Put the arm on the injured side in a sling. Adjust sling so hand is slightly above level of elbow. Tie the arm to the side of the body with triangular, roller or other bandage. Tie snugly but not tight enough to interfere with circulation. You should be able to feel pulse at the wrist after the bandage is in place.

Elbow Fracture

Look for swelling about elbow joint.

What to do

Do not attempt to move arm at the elbow joint if you suspect a fracture in or near the elbow. If arm is either bent or straight, leave it that way.

If the arm is straight, put on a single splint extending from fingertips to armpit. Put the splint on the palm side of the arm. Fasten securely with ties.

If the arm is bent, put the arm in a sling, and bind it firmly to side of body.

Forearm or Wrist Fracture

What to do

Apply a padded splint from palm to elbow.

Support the arm in a sling adjusted so fingers are about 4 inches higher than elbow. Leave fingertips uncovered so they can be watched for signs of swelling or blueness. If these signs appear, carefully loosen splint or sling slightly.

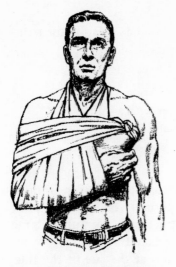

Collarbone Fracture

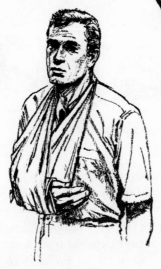

Elbow Fracture

**Forearm or
Wrist Fracture**

Get the victim to doctor as soon as possible for treatment to avoid permanent damage.

FINGER FRACTURE

Immobilize the injured finger with a splint.
Use a sling to support the hand.

KNEECAP FRACTURE

The kneecap, or patella, a small bone just in front of the knee joint, plays an important role in knee joint action. When the patella is fractured, the pull of large leg muscles tends to separate broken fragments.

Look for pain and tenderness at the site of the fracture, inability to straighten out injured leg. Sometimes gentle running of fingers over kneecap will disclose a groove due to separation of the bony fragments.

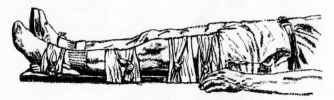

Kneecap Fracture

What to do

Gently straighten out the leg.

Best splint is a strong board, 4 to 6 inches wide, long enough to reach from buttock to just below heel. Pad well with clean rags or other material. Tie limb to board, leaving kneecap itself exposed since there may be rapid swelling. Check every 20–30 minutes to see that bindings do not cut off circulation. Loosen slightly if necessary.

If no board is available, place pillow or rolled-up blanket under knee and tie in place.

Transport victim lying down.

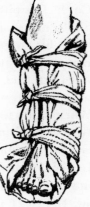

Foot or Toe Fracture

FOOT OR TOE FRACTURE

What to do

Remove shoe and sock quickly since swelling may be rapid. Cut off shoe and sock if necessary.

Apply dressings padded with cotton, or a small pillow, and bandage in place snugly.

Frostbite

Frostbite involves freezing of a part of the body, usually small, but occasionally extensive. Nose, ears, cheeks, fingers and toes are among areas affected most often.

Just prior to frostbite, the skin may be slightly pink. As frostbite develops, it changes to white or greyish-yellow. Blisters may appear later. Pain is sometimes felt early but then subsides. Often, there is no pain; the part feels intensely cold and numb. The victim may not be aware of frostbite until he or someone else observes the glossy skin.

What to do

Cover frostbitten area with warm hand or woolen cloth. If fingers or hand are frostbitten, have victim hold hand in his armpit.

Bring victim indoors as soon as possible.

Put frostbitten part in lukewarm water. If this is not practical, gently warm the part in blankets.

When part is warmed, encourage victim to move it.

Give warm drink (not alcoholic).

Get early medical attention.

DO NOT use hot water, hot water bottles, or heat lamps over a frostbitten area. DO NOT rub with ice or snow; DO NOT rub at all. Rubbing appears to increase risk of gangrene.

Heartbeat Irregularities

PREMATURE HEARTBEATS

Premature beats—or extra-systoles—are common, usually have no serious significance but may cause discomfort and anxiety. They may appear without any obvious cause although in some people they may be triggered by smoking, coffee, alcohol or a digestive upset.

Symptoms include chest discomfort, sometimes a slight choking sensation. They're induced when a heartbeat comes too soon and there is then a momentary "skip" succeeded by an extra strong beat. The irregularity may be detected by feeling the pulse at the wrist.

What to do

No first-aid measures usually are needed beyond re-assurance, explanation. A glass of cold water often makes the victim feel better.

If condition persists, a physician should be seen.

RAPID HEARTBEAT

While exercise or excitement predictably makes the heart beat faster, the heart suddenly may start to beat very rapidly without apparent cause. It may resume normal beating just as suddenly. Known as paroxysmal tachycardia, the condition may indicate an underlying heart trouble but more often doesn't.

Symptoms may include chest discomfort (often a "fluttering" sensation); dizziness; faintness; sometimes, actual fainting. Pulse rate may be 120 or more per minute.

What to do

Make the victim as comfortable as possible. Reassure.

If the rapid beating doesn't subside, bending forward or holding the breath may help.

If condition persists, a physician should be called.

Heat Cramps

Usually involving abdominal muscles or limb muscles, heat cramps may follow profuse perspiration and loss of salt.

What to do

Firm pressure rather than vigorous kneading helps provide relief.

Warm, wet towels add to comfort.

In addition, give salt-water solution (1 teaspoon salt to 1 quart water).

Heat Exhaustion

Symptoms include: pale, clammy skin; weak, rapid pulse; weakness, headache or nausea; sometimes dizziness, vomiting. Heat cramps may accompany heat exhaustion.

What to do

Lay victim down with head level or lower than rest of body.

Give salt-water solution (1 teaspoon salt to 1 quart of water). Have him drink several glasses if he can.

If possible, move victim to cool place but protect from chilling.

Heat Stroke

Symptoms include: hot, flushed skin; rapid pulse. There may be dizziness and nausea. Unconsciousness occurs in severe cases. Temperature is high—often 106, sometimes above 109. Heat stroke is extremely dangerous.

What to do

A physician is urgently needed. Meanwhile:

Sponge body freely with cool water or use cold applications. Try to reduce temperature to more tolerable levels—about 103. (If you have no thermometer, a pulse rate below 110 per minute offers some indication of tolerable temperature.) At this point, stop sponging for 10 minutes, observe victim. If temperature starts to rise again, renew sponging.

If victim is conscious and able to swallow, give salt-water solution (1 teaspoon salt to 1 quart water).

Hernia

A hernia or rupture is the protrusion of a piece of bowel through a weak place in the abdominal muscular wall. Hernias occur in both sexes but are more common in men.

About 80 percent of ruptures occur through the inguinal region or groin. Another weak point is on each side low in the abdomen.

A painful swelling may appear suddenly. Size may be anywhere in the range from small marble to doubled-up fist. The swelling is likely to appear after heavy lifting, pushing, coughing.

What to do

Do not try to push or manipulate the protruding piece of bowel causing the swelling back into place. Serious damage may result.

Have the victim lie flat on his back, with knees drawn up. This may allow the loop of bowel to return to the abdomen.

If this fails, have the victim turn over on his stomach and bring knees up under chest so buttocks are raised, remaining in this position for several minutes.

If the hernia still has not been reduced, have the victim lie on his back again, and apply cold compresses to hernia site. Get a physician. A piece of bowel may be caught in the hernia opening, requiring immediate medical attention. If the victim must be transported, use a stretcher.

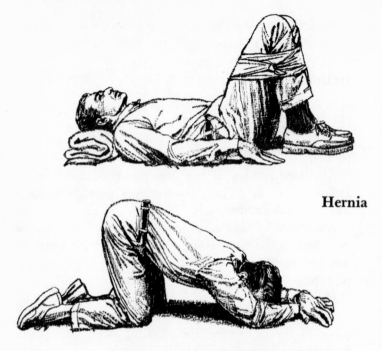

Hernia

If the hernia has been successfully reduced, apply cold compresses. Since the hernia may slip out again, activities on the trail should be reduced to the minimum. The victim should consult a physician upon return home if not before.

Hiccups

Commonly the result of eating too rapidly or, too much, drinking alcoholic beverages, or indigestion, hiccups usually are mild and fleeting.
What to do
Have the victim hold his breath as long as he can.

If this fails to stop the hiccups, have the victim gently pull his tongue as far out of his mouth as he can and hold it extended for a minute or two.

Another measure that sometimes works: Drinking a glass of cold water or cold water containing half a teaspoon of baking soda.

If the hiccups still persist, try the paper bag maneuver. Have victim place bag tightly over nose and mouth and breathe in and out of it for a minute or two so he rebreathes his exhaled carbon dioxide.

Insect Bites and Stings

BEE OR WASP

Remove stinger with tweezers.

Apply a paste made of baking soda and cold cream, if available.

Cold cloths will help relieve pain.

Itching may be relieved by application of calamine lotion.

NOTE: Such measures suffice for ordinary bee or wasp stings. But an insect sting can endanger the life of a person who has become sensitized. Any person who has experienced unusually severe local reactions or generalized allergic reactions in the past should receive desensitization treatment from a physician before risking exposure to a sting.

In case a sting victim experiences an unusual reaction or has a history of severe reaction in the past, do the following:

1. Use a constricting bandage on arm or leg above a

sting. Wrap a strong, wide piece of cloth around the limb. Tie a half-knot, put a short stick on top of half-knot; tie a full knot over stick. Twist the stick. After twisting, there should still be a pulse below the bandage and the bandage should not be so tight as to produce a throbbing sensation. Loosen bandage for a few seconds every 15 minutes.

2. Apply ice pack or cold cloths to area.

3. Rush to doctor as soon as possible.

CHIGGER AND RED BUG BITES

Apply calamine lotion or a paste made of baking soda and small amount of water to relieve itching and discomfort.

TICKS

Small, insect-like creatures about ¼-inch long, ticks cling to grass, leaves, or branches until they can attach themselves to a passing animal or person. They then make a tiny puncture and feed by sucking blood.

While only a small proportion of ticks carry diseases they can transmit to man, there is no feasible way to tell which do and which don't.

If you're in a tick-infested area, always examine body and clothes after any exposure. Check the entire body, with particular attention to head, neck, arms, other hairy areas. Ticks may not be felt even when they are feeding on you. It's important to remove them promptly since disease germs may not be transmitted for as long as 6 hours after ticks attach themselves and begin to feed.

In removing a tick, be careful not to crush since it

Removing Tick

may be loaded with germs. Remove with tweezers. Don't jerk; the mouth may break off and remain embedded in skin. Pull off gently. If the tick clings, hold a lighted cigarette or heated needle to its posterior until it lets go. Or cover it with a drop of oil or turpentine and pull gently.

After removal, gently scrub area with soap and water. Sterilize tweezers by boiling.

Poison Ivy, Oak and Sumac

At the first sign of redness and itching, wash skin with hot water and soap (laundry soap is most effective in cutting the poisonous oils) or a detergent. NOTE: Omit washing if large blisters have begun to appear.

Lessen itching and burning by applying calamine lotion.

If calamine is not available, make a paste of melted soap and water—about lard consistency—and apply thickly. Let dry. Allow to remain on overnight.

Snow Blindness

Symptoms include: burning, smarting of eyes; pain in eyes or forehead; sensitivity to light.
What to do
Apply cold compresses on eyes.
Use mild eye drops or mineral oil.
Wear dark glasses.

Sprains

Sprains are injuries to soft tissues surrounding joints. Ligaments, muscle tendons and blood vessels are stretched, sometimes torn or partially torn. Ankles, fingers, wrists and knees are most commonly affected.

Symptoms include: swelling, tenderness and pain on motion. Sometimes, skin over a large area may become discolored because of rupture of small blood vessels.
What to do
If there is any possibility of fracture as well as sprain, splint the part and treat as you would for fracture (See FRACTURES).

Otherwise—

Rest and elevate the injured part. For ankle sprain, have victim lie down. Place pillows or folded clothing under leg and ankle so ankle is about 12 inches higher than rest of body. For knee sprain, put pillow or padding under leg. For wrist sprain, put arm in sling ad-

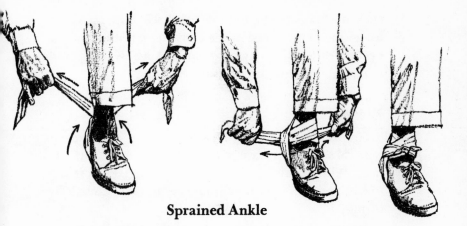

Sprained Ankle

justed so fingers are about 4 inches higher than elbow. For elbow sprain, also put arm in sling.

Apply cold compresses to injured joint. This helps contract blood vessels, minimizes leakage of blood, tends to reduce swelling and pain. Continue cold applications until doctor can be reached. (All sprains should be X-rayed for possible fractures.) If doctor cannot be reached until a day or so after injury, change cold applications to hot compresses or hot water bottle after 24 hours. Do not use heat immediately after injury when it will increase leakage from blood vessels. Later, when blood clotting seals off any damaged vessels, heat is useful.

If there is no other way and the victim of a sprained ankle must walk on it, do this: Loosen shoe laces to allow for swelling but do not remove shoes. Place the middle of a bandage (preferably a folded triangular one) under shoe just in front of heel. Carry bandage ends up and back, crossing them above the heel. Bring ends forward and cross them over instep. Then carry ends downward and toward the heel. Slip each end under the loop formed in the early steps, just in front of heel on each side, carrying them back across instep and tying securely with square knot.

Strains

Strains are injuries to muscles because of overexertion. Muscle fibers are stretched, sometimes partially torn. While strains can occur in any muscle, most frequent are those in back muscles, usually caused by lifting.

Symptoms include: sharp pain or cramp at time of injury; stiffness and pain on movement which may increase within a few hours; some swelling of affected muscle.

What to do

Have victim rest injured area, sitting or lying quietly in comfortable position.

Apply hot compresses.

Massage gently—in the direction of the heart—to stimulate blood flow in that direction. Gentle massage may help lessen stiffness.

Sunstroke (See *Heat Stroke*)

Sty

A sty is an eyelid infection caused by organisms growing in the small glands near the lid edge.

It may begin with a "foreign body" sensation. A small, reddish, painful swelling develops on the lid. In a day or so, a small yellowish spot appears in the center of the swelling. Later, the sty ruptures, discharges pus, and there is relief of pain.

What to do

Do not squeeze.

If sty is just developing, it may be halted by applying cold compresses for a 15-minute period every three or four hours.

If sty is further along—with yellowish spot showing—apply hot compresses for 10 minutes at a time three or four times a day.

Toothache

What to do

Check mouth under good light. If no cavity can be seen, apply ice bag or cold compress against the jaw on the affected side. If this does not help, heat sometimes does. Try hot water bottle or other heat application.

If a cavity is visible, clean it out gently with sterile cotton on the end of a toothpick. Then saturate another tiny bit of sterile cotton with oil of cloves and pack it gently into cavity with toothpick. Be careful not to let oil of cloves touch tongue or inside of mouth; it burns. If packing does not provide sufficient relief, add hot or cold applications.

Unconsciousness

Unconsciousness has many possible causes, ranging from skull fracture, blood loss, shock, sunstroke, heat exhaustion, poisoning or stroke to simple fainting.

Get medical help if at all possible.

Of use in distinguishing various types of unconsciousness is the color of the victim's face, which is likely to be red, white or blue.

RED UNCONSCIOUSNESS

Face is red or flushed. Pulse is often strong but slow. In red unconsciousness, there is increased pressure within the skull along with congestion of blood vessels of face leading to flushing. May be the result of stroke or skull injury but may also stem from other injuries.

What to do

Lay the victim down with head raised slightly above the level of the rest of the body.

Give no stimulants. Give nothing at all by mouth while the victim is unconscious; it could lead to choking.

Apply ice bag or cloths wrung out in cold water to the head.

Keep the victim warm with covers.

Move only if essential—and on a stretcher.

WHITE UNCONSCIOUSNESS

Face is pale. Pulse is weak. Skin feels cold, clammy. In white unconsciousness, paleness develops because of a drop in blood pressure. The drop may be the result of hemorrhage, shock or other cause. Simple fainting is the most common type of white unconsciousness.

What to do

Lay victim down with head slightly lower than rest of

body. Rolled-up clothing under hips will help lower head.

Give nothing by mouth while unconsciousness persists.

If there is no evidence of skull injury, it may help to hold aromatic spirits of ammonia under nose.

Cover victim to keep him warm but do not produce sweating.

When victim begins to regain consciousness, recovery may be hastened by giving him half a teaspoon of aromatic spirits of ammonia in half a glass of water.

Move only if essential—and on stretcher.

BLUE UNCONSCIOUSNESS

Face has a bluish tinge. Pulse is weak. Breathing may be irregular or absent. In blue unconsciousness, oxygen supply in blood is low.

What to do

Quickly lay victim down.

If he is not breathing at all or not breathing adequately, begin ARTIFICIAL RESPIRATION at once.

Keep the victim warm.

Wounds

PUNCTURE

A puncture wound is one in which the skin and underlying tissues are penetrated by a sharp object— anything from a nail to a needle, knife point or sliver of wood, metal or glass.

Puncture Wound

Usually the opening at the skin surface is relatively small and bleeding is limited. This increases the risk of infection since the penetrating object pushes and drags germs deep and the small amount of bleeding doesn't help wash them out.

A special danger in a puncture wound is tetanus (lockjaw) infection, easy to prevent but extremely difficult to treat.

What to do

Encourage bleeding by gentle pressure about the wound. Avoid bruising the wound by hard squeezing.

Do not probe into wound. If a large splinter or other object is still there, attempts to remove it may produce severe bleeding.

Wash the wound with soap and water.

Apply sterile pad and bandage.

Have a doctor clean out the wound thoroughly and give a tetanus protective shot if needed.

GUNSHOT

Stop the bleeding (See HEAVY BLEEDING).

Apply sterile pad and bandage.

If any fractures are evident—or suspected—immobilize (see FRACTURE).

Treat for SHOCK (which see).

Get the victim to a doctor as soon as possible for thorough examination, treatment and protection against tetanus.

ABDOMINAL

Wounds of the abdomen must always be considered serious emergencies. With a torn-open abdomen, the intestines may protrude. Even when there is little bleeding to the outside, there may be much bleeding inside. Shock is usually severe.

What to do

Have the victim lie quietly on his back.

Keep him warm.

Give nothing to drink.

Do not attempt to clean wound. Cover it with sterile dressing and bandage.

If the intestines are protruding, don't touch them or try to push them back. Cover immediately with sterile dressing and bandage. Fasten bandage firmly. Keep dressing and bandage moist to prevent severe damage if the intestines dry out. If possible, moisten with warm water that has been previously boiled and to which you add 1 teaspoon of table salt per pint. If this is not possible, use any clean water; it's likely to be safer than allowing drying out of the intestines.

Keep the victim on his back, knees raised by rolled up clothing or blanket. This position helps keep the abdominal wall relaxed, reducing tendency for intestines to protrude.

Transport to doctor or hospital as quickly as possible —on a stretcher—making certain he remains lying down.

Transporting Victims

Do not needlessly rush to move a seriously injured person.

If at all possible, first aid should be rendered—bleeding controlled, breathing maintained, any suspected fracture sites splinted—before moving.

But if there is urgent need to get the victim away from the accident site at once because of danger of further injury if he is left there, then you may have to pull or lift him to safety.

In pulling: Pull head or feet first, not sideways.

In lifting: If lifting must be done before a check can be made for injuries, support every part of the body, keeping it in as straight a line as possible.

Long Haul

Transporting an injured or ill person for long distances under backwoods conditions is never easy. Great care is needed to avoid making injury or shock worse and aggravating existing illness.

Consider every possibility of getting medical help to the scene or of helicopter evacuation: If there is no such possibility, follow these guidelines:

Stretcher: This is the best means for transporting a seriously injured or ill person. A folding type canvas or metal cot can be used. Or a stretcher can be improvised by buttoning a coat or several shirts over two sturdy branches, or by wrapping a blanket about the branches or poles.

Preparations: Before transporting, give as much first aid as possible. Make the victim as comfortable as pos-

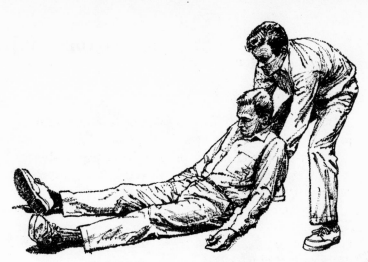

Dragging Victim Head First

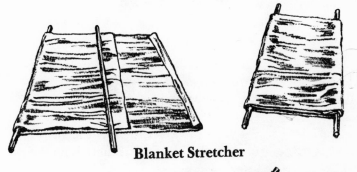

Blanket Stretcher

Coat Stretcher
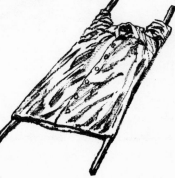

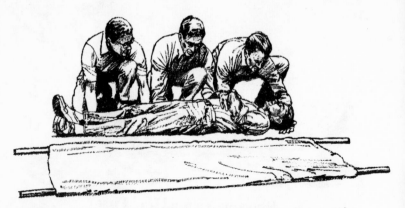

Loaders should be on victim's uninjured side, all kneeling
on knee nearest victim's feet.

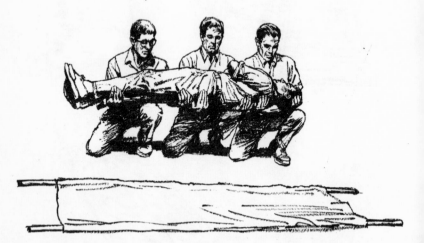

At command "Lift," loaders raise victim gently to their
knees.

PERSON ONTO A STRETCHER

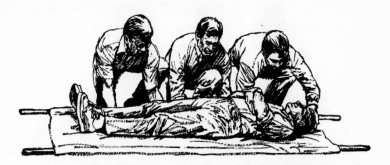

Loader in command moves stretcher under victim and he is lowered to stretcher.

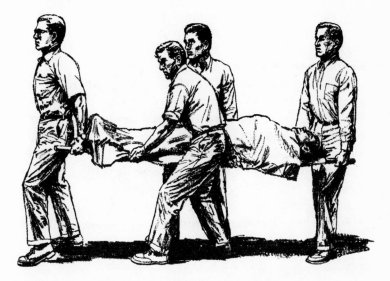

Victim is covered and tied to stretcher. If possible, there should be a bearer at each end and at each side.

sible. Loosen any tight clothing. Treat victim for shock.

Loading: Ideally, at least three people should load and unload a stretcher.

Victim should be on his back, feet tied if possible. Place stretcher close.

Loaders should position themselves facing victim's uninjured side—one at shoulder level, one at hips, the third at the feet. All should kneel on the knee nearest victim's feet. Arms should be positioned under victim— at neck, shoulder, back, thighs, legs, feet. One loader should give the command "Lift," and all together should bring the victim up on their knees. Loader in command should move stretcher in under victim, then signal to lower him gently on stretcher.

Cover victim. See that any needed padding is in place. Tie victim to stretcher as comfortably as possible—and securely enough to prevent slippage and rolling.

Carrying: In addition to one bearer at each end, there should be one on each side if possible.

Victim should be carried so he can see where he is going. Usually, his head should be a little lower than the rest of his body unless breathing is difficult or the head has been injured. If the injury is to the back of the head, victim should be on his side.

Keep a close watch for any signs of increasing shock. Treat.

Periodically check dressings. Adjust if necessary.

Unloading: Reverse the procedure used for loading.

INDEX

Index

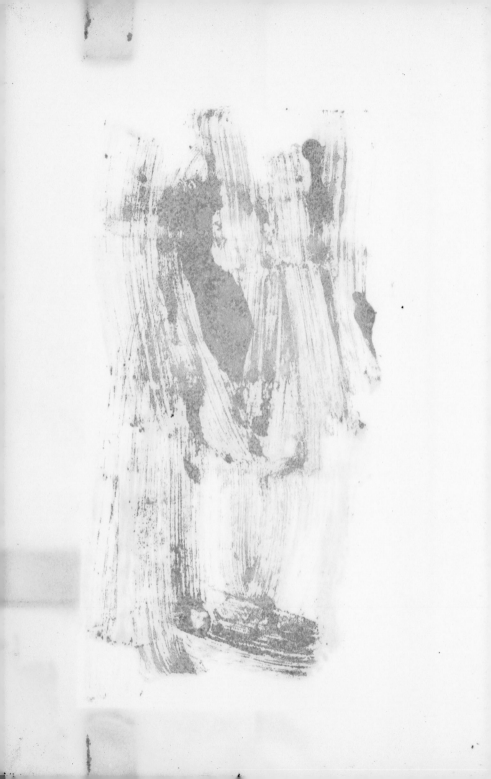